Histological Typing of Lung and Pleural Tumours

Springer
Berlin
Heidelberg
New York
Barcelona
Hong Kong
London
Milan
Paris
Singapore
Tokyo

World Health Organization

The series *International Histological Classification of Tumours* consists of the following volumes. Each of these volumes – apart from volumes 1 and 2, which have already been revised – will appear in a revised edition within the next few years. Volumes of the current editions can be ordered through WHO, Distribution and Sales, Avenue Appia, CH-1211 Geneva 27.

A coded compendium of the International Histological Classification of Tumours (1978).

Histological Typing of Lung and Pleural Tumours

W. D. Travis, T. V. Colby, B. Corrin
Y. Shimosato, and E. Brambilla

In Collaboration with L.H. Sobin
and Pathologists from 14 Countries

Third Edition

With 150 Colour Figures

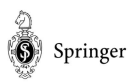 Springer

W. D. Travis
Department of Pulmonary
and Mediastinal Pathology,
Armed Forces Institute of Pathology,
Washington, DC, 20306–6000 USA

T. V. Colby
Department of Pathology,
Mayo Clinic, Scottsdale;
AZ 85259, USA

B. Corrin
Department of Histopathology,
Royal Brompton Hospital,
Sydney Street, London SW3 6NP, UK

Y. Shimosato
Visiting Professor, Keio University
School of Medicine, Shinanomachi,
Shinjukuku, Tokyo 160–0016, Japan

E. Brambilla
Service de Pathologie Cellulaire,
Centre Hospitalier Universitaire
de Grenoble, B.P. 217–38043,
Grenoble, France

L. H. Sobin
Head, WHO Collaborating Center
for the International Histological
Classification of Tumours
Armed Forces Institute of Pathology
Washington, DC 20306-6000, USA

First edition published by WHO in 1967. Second edition published by WHO in 1981

ISBN 3-540-65219-1 Springer Verlag Berlin Heidelberg New York

Cataloging-in-Publication Data applied for

Die Deutsche Bibliothek – Cip-Einheitsaufnahme
Histological typing of lung and pleural tumours / W. D. Travis ...
in collab. with L. H. Sobin and pathologists from 14 countries. –
Berlin ; Heidelberg ; New York ; Barcelone ; Hong Kong ; London ;
Milan ; Paris ; Singapore ; Tokyo : Springer, 1999
    ISBN 3-540-65219-1

© Springer-Verlag Berlin Heidelberg 1999
Printed in Germany

The use of general descriptive names, registered names, trademarks, etc. in this publication does not imply, even in the absence of a specific statement, that such names are exempt from the relevant protective laws and regulations and therefore free for general use.

Product liability: The publisher cannot guarantee the accuracy of any information about dosage and application contained in this book. In every individual case the user must check such information by consulting the relevant literature.

Typesetting and Production: Pro Edit GmbH, Heidelberg, Germany
Printing, and bookbinding: Konrad Triltsch, Druck- und Verlagsanstalt GmbH, Würzburg, Germany

SPIN: 10699005   81/3135 – 5 4 3 2 1 0 – Printed on acid-free paper

Participants

Pathology Panels of the World Health Organization and the International Association for the Study of Lung Cancer

Chair WHO Panel

Travis, W.D., Dr.
Department of Pulmonary and Mediastinal Pathology,
Armed Forces Institute of Pathology,
Washington, DC, 20306–6000 USA

Chair IASLC Panel

Hirsch, F.R., Dr.
Copenhagen, Denmark

Coordinators

Colby, T.V., Dr.
Department of Pathology, Mayo Clinic,
Scottsdale, AZ USA

Corrin, B., Dr.
Department of Histopathology, Royal Brompton Hospital,
London, UK

Shimosato, Y., Dr.
Visiting Professor, Keio University School of Medicine,
Tokyo, Japan

Brambilla, E., Dr.
Service de Pathologie Cellulaire, Centre Hospitalier Universitaire
de Grenoble, Grenoble, France

Core Panel Members

Alvarez-Fernandez, E., Dr.
Madrid, Spain

Hammar, S.P., Dr.
Bremerton, WA, USA

Hasleton, P.S., Dr.
Manchester, UK

Mackay, B., Dr.
Houston, TX, USA

Popper, H., Dr.
Graz, Austria

Steele, R.H., Dr.
Woolloongabba, Australia

Contribution on preinvasive lesions by Wilbur Franklin, MD, Denver, CO, USA; Chair, International Association for the Study of Lung Cancer (IASLC)/National Cancer Institute SPORE Pathology Working Group for Classification of Preinvasive Epithelial Abnormalities of Lung
The panel chairs and coordinators are also core panel members and IASLC pathology panel members.

Extended Panel of Reviewers

*Aisner, S., Dr.**
Newark, NJ, USA

Churg, A., Dr.
Vancouver, British Columbia, Canada

Dehner, L.P., Dr.
St. Louis, MO, USA

*Gazdar, A.F., Dr.**
Dallas, TX, USA

Henderson, D.W., Dr.
Bedford Park, South Australia

Jambhekar, N.A., Dr.
Parel Bombay, India

Koss, M.N., Dr.
Los Angeles, CA, USA

Müller, K.M., Dr.
Bochum, Germany

Petrovitchev, N., Dr.
Moscow, Russia

Saldiva, P., Dr.
Sao Paulo, Brazil

Sheppard, M., Dr.
London, UK

Wagenaar, Sj. Sc. Dr.
Amsterdam, The Netherlands

Li, Wei-hua, Dr.
Beijing, P.R. China

---

* IASLC Pathology Panel members.

General Preface to the Series

Among the prerequisites for comparative studies of cancer are international agreement on histological criteria for the definition and classification of cancer types and a standardized nomenclature. An internationally agreed classification of tumours, acceptable to physicians, surgeons, radiologists, pathologists and statisticians alike, would enable cancer workers in all parts of the world to compare their findings and would facilitate collaboration among them.

In a report published in 1952[1], a subcommittee of the World Health Organization (WHO) Expert Committee on Health Statistics discussed the general principles that should govern the statistical classification of tumours and agreed that, to ensure the necessary flexibility and ease of coding, three separate classifications were needed according to (1) anatomical site, (2) histological type and (3) degree of malignancy. A classification according to anatomical site is available in the International Classification of Diseases[2].

In 1956, the WHO Executive Board passed a resolution[3] requesting the Director-General to explore the possibility that WHO might organize centres in various parts of the world and arrange for the collection of human tissues and their histological classification. The main purpose of such centres would be to develop histological definitions of cancer types and to facilitate the wide adoption of a uniform nomenclature. The resolution was endorsed by the Tenth World Health Assembly in May 1957[4].

---

[1] WHO (1952) WHO Technical Report Series, no. 53. WHO, Geneva, p 45
[2] WHO (1952) WHO Technical Report Series, no. 53. WHO, Geneva, p 45
  WHO (1977) Manual of the international statistical classification of diseases, injuries, and causes of death. WHO, Geneva
[3] WHO (1956) WHO Official Records, no. 68, p 14 (resolution EB 17.R40)
[4] WHO (1957) WHO Official Records, no. 79, p 467 (resolution WHA 10.18)

Since 1958, WHO has established a number of centres concerned with this subject. The result of this endeavor has been the *International Histological Classification of Tumours*, a multivolumed series published from 1967 onwards. The present volume aims to update the classification, reflecting progress in diagnosis and the relevance of tumour types to clinical and epidemiological features.

Preface to Histological Typing of Lung and Pleural Tumours, Third Edition

The first edition of *Histological Typing of Lung Tumours* was published in 1967[5]. It was revised in 1981[6]. The pathology panel of the International Association for the Study of Lung Cancer was selected by the WHO to prepare the revised classification. The panel was divided into a core group, which participated in several discussion meetings and an extended panel of reviewers, all of whom reviewed drafts of the proposed classification. The members of the core group and extended panel of reviewers are listed on pp. V-VIII. The histological classification listed on pp. 21-24 contains the morphology codes of the *International Classification of Diseases for Oncology* (ICD-O)[7] and the *Systematized Nomenclature of Medicine* (SNOMED)[8].

It should be appreciated that the classification of tumours of the lung and pleura reflects the current state of knowledge, and that modifications are certain to be needed as more information is accumulated. Nevertheless, it is hoped that, in the interests of international cooperation, all pathologists will use the classification as proposed.

The publications in the series *International Histological Classification of Tumours* are not intended to serve as textbooks, but rather to promote the adoption of a uniform terminology that will facilitate communication among cancer workers. For this reason, literature references have intentionally been largely omitted and readers should refer to standard works for bibliographies.

The editors and authors are grateful to the International Association for the Study of Lung Cancer for its generous financial support.

[5] World Health Organization (1967) Histological typing of lung tumours, 1st edn. WHO, Geneva

[6] World Health Organization (1981) Histological typing of lung tumors, 2nd edn. WHO, Geneva

[7] World Health Organization (1990) International classification of diseases for oncology, 2nd edn. WHO, Geneva

[8] College of American Pathologists (1982) Systematized nomenclature of medicine. College of American Pathologists, Chicago

Acknowledgements. We would like to gratefully acknowledge the International Association for the Study of Lung Cancer (IASLC) for allowing their pathology panel to serve as the primary members of the committee to formulate this classification. We also thank the IASLC for providing the funding for the WHO committee meetings and for supporting the work of the IASLC Pathology Panel that led to the selection for this project.

We would also like to gratefully acknowledge Ms. Robin-Anne Ferris and Mr. Richard Dreyfus for outstanding assistance with photography. Thanks also go to Dr. Douglas B. Flieder, for contributing photographs of endometriosis and papillomas, to Dr. Ernest Lack for contributing the case of pulmonary chondroma, to Dr. John K. Chan for contributing the case of lymphoepithelial-like carcinoma, and to Dr. Andrew Nicholson for contributing the case of bronchial inflammatory polyp and inverted squamous papillomas. We also thank Drs. R.C. Curran and E.L. Jones for contributing the lung teratoma for photography.

Contents

Introduction

Lung cancer is currently the most frequently diagnosed major cancer in the world and the most common cause of cancer mortality worldwide. This is largely due to the carcinogenic effects of cigarette smoke. Over the coming decades, changes in smoking habits will greatly influence lung cancer incidence and mortality throughout the world. These changes may also impact upon the histological types of lung cancer.

Tumour classification is important for consistency in patient treatment, and because it provides a basis for epidemiologic and biological studies.

The previous WHO classification was published in 1981 and since then considerable progress has been made in our understanding of certain lung tumours[1]. The concept of neuroendocrine tumours of the lung has been refined with recognition of large cell neuroendocrine carcinoma and modification of criteria for atypical carcinoid. Atypical adenomatous hyperplasia is now recognized as a potential precursor to adenocarcinoma. Studies have documented the histological heterogeneity of lung carcinomas, particularly among adenocarcinomas and poorly differentiated carcinomas. Molecular studies have also shown that hamartomas and sclerosing hemangiomas are true neoplasms rather than tumour-like lesions.

This classification is based on histological characteristics of tumours seen in surgical or needle biopsy and autopsy material. Though a large percentage of lung carcinomas are now diagnosed on cytology specimens, the classification does not address cytology.

The definitions of the tumour types in this book are based primarily on light microscopy in order to achieve the widest application throughout the world and so that comparability of data will be feasible and consistent. Ancillary techniques (histochemistry, immunohistochemistry), electron microscopy, tissue culture and molecular biol-

---

[1] World Health Organization (1981) Histological typing of lung tumors, 2nd edn. WHO, Geneva

Table 1. Microscopic features of squamous dysplasia and carcinoma in situ (continued on page 3)

Abnormality	Thickness	Cell size	Maturation/orientation	Nuclei
Mild dysplasia	Mildly increased	Mildly increased Mild anisocytosis, pleomorphism	Continuous progression of maturation from base to luminal surface Basilar zone expanded with cellular crowding in lower third Distinct intermediate (prickle cell) zone present Superficial flattening of epithelial cells	Mild variation of N/C ratio Finely granular chromatin Minimal angulation Nucleoli inconspicuous or absent Nuclei vertically oriented in lower third Mitoses absent or very rare
Moderate dysplasia	Moderately increased	Mild increase in cell size; cells often small May have moderate anisocytosis, pleomorphism	Partial progression of maturation from base to luminal surface Basilar zone expanded with cellular crowding in lower two thirds of epithelium Intermediate zone confined to upper third of epithelium Superficial flattening of epithelial cells	Moderate variation of N/C ratio Finely granular chromatin Angulations, grooves and lobulations present Nucleoli inconspicuous or absent Nuclei vertically oriented in lower two thirds Mitotic figures present in lower third

Table 1. Microscopic features of squamous dysplasia and carcinoma in situ (continued from page 2)

Abnormality	Thickness	Cell size	Maturation/orientation	Nuclei
Severe dysplasia	Markedly increased	Markedly increased May have marked anisocytosis, pleomorphism	Little progression of maturation from base to luminal surface Basilar zone expanded with cellular crowding well into upper third Intermediate zone greatly attenuated Superficial flattening of epithelial cells	N/C ratio often high and variable Chromatin coarse and uneven Nuclear angulations and folding prominent Nucleoli frequently present and conspicuous Nuclei vertically oriented in lower two thirds Mitotic figures present in lower two thirds
Carcinoma in situ	May or may not be increased	May be markedly increased May have marked anisocytosis, pleomorphism	No progression of maturation from base to luminal surface; epithelium could be inverted with little change in appearance Basilar zone expanded with cellular crowding throughout epithelium Intermediate zone absent Surface flattening confined to the most superficial cells	N/C ratio often high and variable Chromatin coarse and uneven Nuclear angulations and folding prominent Nucleoli may be present or inconspicuous No consistent orientation of nuclei in relation to epithelial surface Mitotic figures present through full thickness

N/C = nuclear to cytoplasmic ratio.

ogy can provide valuable information on carcinogenesis, histogenesis and differentiation. It is hoped that those with access to advanced techniques will continue to apply them. However, criteria in the present classification are designed to categorize most tumours largely by conventional methods.

The term "tumour" is used synonymously with neoplasm in this classification. The phrase "tumour-like" is applied to lesions that clinically or morphologically resemble neoplasms but which are not considered to be neoplasms biologically. They are included here because they may be confused with tumours and because of the ill-defined distinction between some neoplasms and certain non-neoplastic lesions. Time-honoured terms have generally been retained to preserve as much continuity with the previous classification as possible, unless there has been a fundamental change in the understanding of a tumour. Synonyms are included only if they have been widely used or if they are considered to be helpful in the understanding of the lesions.

The present classification does not appear as "simple" as those used in the earlier editions. This reflects the increasing information that has become available over the years. For comparisons with earlier data readers can easily "collapse" the various subtypes into the major categories, e.g. squamous cell carcinoma, small cell carcinoma, adenocarcinoma and large cell carcinoma.

Preinvasive Lesions

Compared with the two previous editions[2,3] more precise guidelines for grading squamous dysplasia and carcinoma in situ are provided (Table 1, p. 2 and 3). Two categories have been added to the group of preinvasive lesions: atypical adenomatous hyperplasia and diffuse idiopathic pulmonary neuroendocrine cell hyperplasia.

Studies have implicated atypical adenomatous hyperplasia as a precursor to adenocarcinoma, and this lesion can be difficult to separate from the non-mucinous variant of bronchioloalveolar carcinoma.

While virtually all pulmonary neuroendocrine cell hyperplasias are secondary to airway fibrosis and/or inflammation, a rare disorder

---

[2] World Health Organization (1967) Histological typing of lung tumours, 1st edn. WHO, Geneva

[3] World Health Organization (1981) Histological typing of lung tumors, 2nd edn. WHO, Geneva

Table 2. The spectrum of neuroendocrine (NE) proliferations and neoplasms

I. NE cell hyperplasia and tumourlets	A. NE cell hyperplasia (1) NE cell hyperplasia associated with fibrosis and/or inflammation (2) NE cell hyperplasia adjacent to carcinoid tumours (3) Diffuse idiopathic NE cell hyper plasia with or without airway fibrosis/obstruction B. Tumourlets
II. Tumours with NE morphology	A. Typical carcinoid B. Atypical carcinoid C. Large cell neuroendocrine carcinoma D. Small cell carcinoma
III. Non-small-cell carcinomas with NE differentiation	
IV. Other tumours with NE properties	A. Pulmonary blastoma B. Primitive neuroectodermal tumour C. Desmoplastic round cell tumour D. Carcinomas with rhabdoid phenotype E. Paraganglioma

called diffuse idiopathic pulmonary neuroendocrine cell hyperplasia (DIPNECH) may be associated with airway fibrosis and/or obstruction. In this clinical setting the neuroendocrine cell hyperplasia appears to be a precursor to the development of multiple tumourlets and typical or atypical carcinoids (Table 2).

General Principles of Lung Tumour Typing and Grading

In general, lung carcinomas are classified according to the best-differentiated component and graded by the most poorly differentiated component. Therefore, if a tumour is for the most part undifferentiated but contains focal squamous cell carcinoma or adenocarcinoma, it would be classified as a poorly differentiated squamous cell carcinoma or adenocarcinoma. Exceptions to this are small cell carcinoma, pleomorphic carcinoma and carcinosarcoma, all of which are poorly differentiated tumours.

If a squamous cell carcinoma or an adenocarcinoma includes a component of small cell carcinoma, giant and/or spindle cell carcinoma or sarcoma with heterologous elements, it is classified as a combined small cell carcinoma, pleomorphic carcinoma or carcinosarcoma, respectively.

Histological Heterogeneity

Lung cancers frequently show histological heterogeneity: variation in appearance and differentiation from microscopic field to field and from one histological section to the next. Since the 1981 WHO classification was published, several studies have demonstrated this feature. Almost 50% of lung carcinomas exhibit more than one of the major histological types. This fact has important implications for lung tumour classification and must be kept in mind especially when interpreting small biopsies.

The designation of a minimum requirement such as 10% for the adenocarcinoma and squamous cell carcinoma components of adenosquamous carcinoma, or the spindle and/or giant cell carcinoma component of pleomorphic carcinomas is an arbitrary criterion since the extent of histological sampling will influence classification of such tumours. Although these tumours may be suspected on small specimens such as bronchoscopic or needle biopsies, a definitive diagnosis requires a resected specimen. If this problem arises in a resected tumour, additional histological sections may be helpful. Nevertheless, defining a specific percentage for a histological component can be a useful criterion for entities such as adenosquamous carcinoma and pleomorphic carcinoma.

Special Techniques

It is recognized that immunohistochemistry or electron microscopy may detect differentiation that cannot be seen by routine light microscopy and these techniques are occasionally required for precise classification of lung and pleural tumours. For example, large cell neuroendocrine carcinoma and malignant mesothelioma may require appropriate immunohistochemical and/or electron microscopic findings to confirm the diagnosis.

Trends in Histological Types

Squamous cell carcinoma was for many years the most common variety of lung cancer around the world. However, over the past two decades adenocarcinoma has become recognized as the most common lung cancer type in some countries. Whether this trend will be followed in all parts of the world remains to be determined.

The Spectrum of Neuroendocrine Tumours

Neuroendocrine tumours of the lung are a distinct subset of tumours, which share certain morphologic, ultrastructural, immunohistochemical and molecular characteristics. The major categories of morphologically identifiable neuroendocrine tumours are small cell carcinoma (SCLC), large cell neuroendocrine carcinoma (LCNEC), typical carcinoid and atypical carcinoid (Tables 2 and 3, pp. 5 and 8). Consideration was given to a conceptual grouping of these tumours in this classification. However, because of differences in incidence, clinical, epidemiologic, histologic, survival and molecular characteristics, they are discussed as a spectrum in this introduction, but are categorized separately in the actual classification.

SCLC is maintained as a separate major histological type (see Sect. 1.3.2) for several reasons. SCLC is relatively common, accounting for 15%–25% of all lung malignancies, while typical and atypical carcinoids and LCNEC collectively make up only 2%–3%. SCLC is also the most clinically distinctive of the major types of lung cancer. Its biologic characteristics and responsiveness to chemotherapy sharply distinguish it from most non-small cell carcinomas (NSCLC).

The terms typical and atypical carcinoid are retained for a number of reasons. They share a distinctive basic microscopic appearance and morphologically look like carcinoids found at other body sites. Spindle cell, oncocytic and melanocytic patterns, as well as stromal ossification, occur in both typical and atypical carcinoids. Patients with typical and atypical carcinoids are also significantly younger than those with SCLC and LCNEC. Approximately 20%–40% of patients with both typical and atypical carcinoids are non-smokers, while virtually all patients with SCLC and LCNEC are cigarette smokers. In contrast to SCLC and LCNEC, both typical and atypical carcinoids can occur in patients with multiple endocrine neoplasia (MEN) type I. In

Table 3. Criteria for diagnosis of neuroendocrine (NE) tumours

Typical carcinoid	A tumour with carcinoid morphology and less than two mitoses per 2 mm² (ten HPF[a]), lacking necrosis and 0.5 cm or larger
Atypical carcinoid	A tumour with carcinoid morphology with 2–10 mitoses per 2 mm² (ten HPF[a]) *or* necrosis (often punctate)
Large cell neuroendocrine carcinoma	(1) A tumour with a neuroendocrine morphology (organoid nesting, palisading, rosettes, trabeculae) (2) High mitotic rate: 11 or greater per 2 mm² (ten HPF[a]), median of 70 per 2 mm² (ten HPF[a]) (3) Necrosis (often large zones) (4) Cytologic features of a NSCLC: large cell size, low nuclear to cytoplasmic ratio, vesicular or fine chromatin, and/or frequent nucleoli. Some tumours have fine nuclear chromatin and lack nucleoli, but qualify as NSCLC because of large cell size and abundant cytoplasm (5) Positive immunohistochemical staining for one or more NE markers (other than neuron specific enolase) and/or NE granules by electron microscopy
Small cell carcinoma	(1) Small size (generally less than the diameter of three small resting lymphocytes) (2) Scant cytoplasm (3) Nuclei: finely granular nuclear chromatin, absent or faint nucleoli (4) High mitotic rate (11 or greater per 2 mm² (ten HPF[a]), median of 80 per 2 mm² (ten HPF[a]) (5) Frequent necrosis often in large zones

[a]See explanation of HPF (high power field) area and mitosis counting in Introduction, p. 10.
NSCLC = non-small-cell carcinoma.

addition, neuroendocrine cell hyperplasia with or without tumourlets is relatively frequent in both typical and atypical carcinoids but not in LCNEC or SCLC. Histological heterogeneity with other major histological types of lung carcinoma occurs with both SCLC and LCNEC, but not with typical or atypical carcinoids. In contrast to LCNEC, most typical and atypical carcinoids are readily diagnosed by light microscopy without the need for special tests.

The criteria for atypical carcinoid defined by Arrigoni et al.[3] were fairly specific, especially regarding the level of mitotic activity. How-

---

[3] Arrigoni MG, Woolner LB, Bernatz PE (1972) Atypical carcinoid tumors of the lung. J Thorac Cardiovasc Surg 64:413–421

ever, failure to adhere to these criteria and a proliferation of alternative terms has led to considerable confusion. Of all of the studies on this subject, the criteria proposed by Arrigoni et al. provided the clearest definition of a neuroendocrine tumour of intermediate grade that is readily separable from LCNEC. An argument against use of the term atypical carcinoid is that clinicians and surgeons fail to recognize the aggressive potential of this tumour because the word "carcinoid" is retained. However, all carcinoids are malignant and the significantly worse survival rate of patients with atypical carcinoids has been demonstrated in numerous papers, including Arrigoni's original article. Pathology reports should therefore stress the clinical implications of a diagnosis of atypical carcinoid. In addition, it is not clear that atypical carcinoids respond to therapy other than surgery. While patients with advanced-stage tumours are sometimes given chemotherapy and/or radiation therapy, the effectiveness of these modalities for atypical carcinoids has not been established in reports of tumours meeting the Arrigoni criteria and clearly separated from LCNEC.

LCNEC and SCLC have been kept separate for several reasons. On clinical and morphologic grounds both SCLC and LCNEC are high-grade tumours and P53 mutations are frequent in both. However, we have elected to continue to classify LCNEC as a subtype of large cell carcinoma until it is proven that the chemotherapy used for SCLC is effective for patients with LCNEC (see Sect. 1.3.4.1). At the present time it is not clear how these patients should be treated.

Tumours with Neuroendocrine Morphology

Tumours of the lung with neuroendocrine morphology by light microscopy encompass a three-grade spectrum of low-grade typical carcinoid, intermediate-grade atypical carcinoid and the high-grade LCNEC and SCLC. All of these tumours share, to varying degrees, neuroendocrine features by light microscopy including organoid nesting, palisading, a trabecular pattern and rosette-like structures. The most important criterion for separating typical carcinoid from atypical carcinoid is mitotic activity. Arrigoni et al.[4] originally proposed that atypical carcinoids had between five and ten mitoses per ten high-power fields. However, the mitotic range for atypical carcinoid was recently modified to between two and ten mitoses per 2 mm^2 (ten high-

---

[4]Arrigoni MG, Woolner LB, Bernatz PE (1972) Atypical carcinoid tumors of the lung. J Thorac Cardiovasc Surg 64:413–421

power fields; see below for mitosis counting method)[5]. A second criterion for atypical carcinoid is necrosis. Cytologic atypia appears to be less reliable as a diagnostic feature.

A mitotic count of eleven or more mitoses per 2 mm^2 (ten high-power fields) is the main criterion for separating LCNEC and SCLC from atypical carcinoid[5]. LCNEC and SCLC usually have very high mitotic rates, with an average of 70–80 per 2 mm^2 (ten high-power fields in some microscope models). LCNEC and SCLC also generally have more extensive necrosis than atypical carcinoid. LCNEC are separated from SCLC using a constellation of criteria, which include larger cell size, abundant cytoplasm, prominent nucleoli, vesicular or coarse chromatin, polygonal rather than fusiform shape, less prominent nuclear molding and less conspicuous deposition of hematoxylin-stained material (DNA) in blood vessel walls. LCNEC cells more closely resemble those of a large cell carcinoma than a carcinoid tumour. Rarely a tumour with carcinoid morphology has a mitotic rate of more than 10 per 2 mm^2 (ten high-power fields), and because it is likely to be particularly aggressive it is best classified as a LCNEC.

Mitoses should be counted in the areas of highest mitotic activity and the fields counted should be filled with as many viable tumour cells as possible. Since the area viewed in a high-power field varies considerably depending on the microscope model, we define the mitotic range based on the area of viable tumour examined. These criteria were established on a microscope with a 40× objective, an eyepiece field-of-view number of 20 and with no magnification changing devices. With this approach the area viewed in one high-power field is 0.2 mm^2 and ten high-power fields equals 2 mm^2. If microscopes with other objective and eyepiece field-of-view numbers are used, the area in a high-power field should be measured to allow calibration to cover a 2 mm^2 area.

The widely variable published terminology and criteria for neuroendocrine lung tumours hinder understanding of this complicated subject. Many terms have been used for neuroendocrine lung tumours, including well-differentiated neuroendocrine carcinoma, neuroendocrine carcinoma (grades 1–3), intermediate cell neuroendocrine carcinoma, malignant carcinoid and peripheral small cell carcinoma resembling carcinoid. All carcinoid tumours are malignant, so the use

---

[5] Travis WD, Rush W, Flieder D, Fleming MV, Gal A, Falk R, Koss MN (1998) Survival analysis of 200 pulmonary neuroendocrine tumors: with clarification of criteria for atypical carcinoid and its separation from typical carcinoid. Am J Surg Pathol 22:934–944

of the term malignant carcinoid implies there is a benign carcinoid and is misleading. Typical carcinoids have an indolent clinical course, and though regional lymph node metastases can be found in up to 15% of cases, they only rarely metastasize distantly and cause death.

It has been shown that there is substantial reproducibility (κ statistic of 0.70) for subclassification of pulmonary neuroendocrine tumours using the classification scheme proposed in Tables 2 and 3 (pp. 5 and 8). The greatest reproducibility is seen with SCLC and typical carcinoid. The most common disagreements involve LCNEC vs SCLC, followed by typical carcinoid vs atypical carcinoid and atypical carcinoid vs LCNEC. More study of the uncommon atypical carcinoid and LCNEC is needed to better define their clinical characteristics and to determine the optimal approach to therapy.

Non-small-cell Carcinomas with Neuroendocrine Differentiation

Some lung carcinomas, which do not show neuroendocrine morphology by light microscopy, demonstrate immunohistochemical and/or ultrastructural evidence of neuroendocrine differentiation. Neuroendocrine differentiation can be shown by immunohistochemistry in 10%–20% percent of squamous cell carcinomas, adenocarcinomas and large cell carcinomas. It is seen most often in adenocarcinomas. These tumours are collectively referred to as "NSCLC with neuroendocrine differentiation" (NSCLC-ND) (see Table 2, p. 5). While this issue has drawn much interest, there is controversy over whether these tumours are associated with worse or better survival rates and whether they are more or less responsive to chemotherapy than NSCLC lacking neuroendocrine differentiation. Therefore, these tumours require further study before they are included as a separate category in a histological classification. They should be classified according to the conventional typing herein, with neuroendocrine differentiation noted.

Electron Microscopy and Immunohistochemical Markers

In sections from paraffin-embedded tissue, a panel of immunohistochemical markers is the best way to detect neuroendocrine differentiation. Chromogranin and synaptophysin are the most reliable markers at the present time. Certain neural cell adhesion molecule (NCAM) antibodies may also be helpful, but neuron-specific enolase is not useful since it stains up to two-thirds of NSCLC.

Neuroendocrine differentiation can be demonstrated by electron microscopy or immunohistochemistry in virtually all typical and atypical carcinoid tumours. However, this is not always true of the high-grade neuroendocrine tumours such as SCLC. Neuroendocrine granules may be absent by electron microscopy in as many as one-third of SCLC and up to 25% of SCLC fail to stain with an immunohistochemical panel of neuroendocrine markers, including chromogranin and synaptophysin. Currently, the diagnosis of LCNEC requires confirmation of neuroendocrine differentiation with either electron microscopy or immunohistochemistry. Large cell carcinomas can express four potential types of neuroendocrine morphology and differentiation detected by special studies: (1) *LCNEC* has both neuroendocrine morphology and differentiation by electron microscopy and/or immunohistochemistry; (2) *large cell carcinomas with neuroendocrine differentiation* lack neuroendocrine morphology but have neuroendocrine markers by electron microscopy or immunohistochemistry; (3) *large cell carcinomas with neuroendocrine morphology* have neuroendocrine morphologic features but lack neuroendocrine markers by electron microscopy or immunohistochemistry; and (4) classic *large cell carcinomas* lack neuroendocrine morphology or differentiation by special studies. Investigations are underway to determine whether there are differences in survival or response to therapy among patients whose large cell carcinomas have these various types of neuroendocrine features.

Adenocarcinoma

Subclassification of adenocarcinoma is fraught with difficulty since these tumours are highly heterogeneous histologically, with only a minority of cases showing a pure histological pattern. The current classification recognizes that most adenocarcinomas will be of the mixed subtype. In such cases the diagnosis should read: "adenocarcinoma, mixed type with components of acinar, papillary, bronchioloalveolar and/or solid with mucin formation", depending on the components identified.

Major changes in the classification of adenocarcinoma from the 1981 WHO proposal[6] include a strict definition of bronchioloalveolar carcinoma and the addition of a mixed type and several variant subtypes. We have restricted bronchioloalveolar carcinoma to non-invasive tumours with lepidic spread. If stromal, vascular or pleural invasion is seen, the tumour is reclassified as adenocarcinoma, mixed type with bronchioloalveolar features. Thus virtually all bronchioloalveolar carcinomas presenting as a solitary mass will be stage I tumours. Liberal sampling of tumours with a bronchioloalveolar pattern will be important in any attempt to exclude the presence of an invasive lesion. On bronchoscopic biopsy, needle biopsy or cytology specimens, a bronchioloalveolar pattern may be recognized, but it will be impossible to make a final histological subclassification since the presence of invasion cannot be excluded. While this is a narrow definition, there is evidence that non-invasive bronchioloalveolar carcinomas of less than 2 cm in size may be curable, while those that are minimally invasive may recur and/or metastasize. Bronchioloalveolar carcinoma is the only subtype of adenocarcinoma with a substantially more favourable prognosis than the other subtypes. We have subclassified bronchioloalveolar carcinoma into mucinous, non-mucinous and mixed subtypes. We also specify that a considerable amount of mucin (five or more cells staining positively for mucin in at least two high-power fields) should be present to diagnose "solid adenocarcinoma with mucin formation" rather than occasional positive cells. This threshold for the amount of mucin is arbitrarily chosen. However, this recommendation was made to discourage the routine use of mucin stains on all lung carcinoma specimens. Mucin stains should only be performed if the presence of mucin is suspected on routine hematoxylin and eosin-stained sections. Stains helpful in demonstrating mucin include mucicarmine and periodic acid–Schiff with diastase digestion.

Further work is needed to better clarify the prognostic significance of adenocarcinoma subtyping based on cases studied with detailed histological criteria.

---

[6] World Health Organization (1981) Histological typing of lung tumors, 2nd edn. WHO, Geneva

Carcinomas with Pleomorphic, Sarcomatoid or Sarcomatous Elements

The classification of carcinomas with pleomorphic, sarcomatoid or sarcomatous elements is problematic and it is difficult to resolve all of the controversial issues in one proposal. For practical reasons we have grouped these tumours (see Sect. 1.3.6) and this relatively simple approach can readily be applied by light microscopy.

The great majority of carcinomas with components of spindle cell and/or giant cell carcinoma are histologically heterogeneous. Pure spindle or giant cell carcinomas are rare. Because of the spindle cells and giant cells, these tumours are often mistaken for sarcomas or carcinosarcomas. Immunohistochemistry and electron microscopy have contributed to an improved understanding of this spectrum of tumours. The spindle and giant cells usually stain with epithelial markers such as keratin, CAM 5.2 and epithelial membrane antigen, but they can be negative. If a component of frank carcinoma is present the tumour is a pleomorphic carcinoma even if epithelial differentiation cannot be proven by special techniques, while the term carcinosarcoma is reserved for tumours with heterologous mesenchymal elements such as malignant bone, cartilage or skeletal muscle. The use of keratin stains is problematic due to difficulties inherent in variable staining methods, interpretation of staining results, and potential staining of both carcinomas and sarcomas. Classification of these tumours is therefore based on light microscopic criteria.

Molecular Biology

Since the 1981 WHO classification[7], molecular biology has made a tremendous impact on the understanding of the genetics of lung cancer. A few of the abnormalities that may be present are mentioned here since they are characteristic of particular histological types of tumours of the lung or pleura.

The accumulation of mutations leading to increased rate of cell division, escape from programmed cell death (apoptosis) and the ability to locally invade and further metastasize, provide the molecular basis

---

[7] World Health Organization (1981) Histological typing of lung tumors, 2nd edn. WHO, Geneva

for neoplasia. This brief review focuses on frequent genetic and molecular abnormalities in lung tumours that are specifically involved in the pathway of carcinogenesis or which could help in distinguishing neoplasia from non-malignant proliferations.

Benign Epithelial Tumours

In a cytogenetic study of one alveolar adenoma, in ten of 54 metaphases studied, a pseudodiploid karyotype, 46,XX,add(16)(q24), was demonstrated. Fluorescence in situ hybridization studies revealed the add(16)(q24) to be a der(16)t(10;16)(q23;q24). This supports the concept that alveolar adenomas are true neoplasms, although this finding needs confirmation in additional studies. Other than this, no frequently occurring and recurrent mutation or molecular abnormality has been described in the various types of adenomas or papillomas of the lung. The presence of the human papilloma virus genome has been demonstrated in squamous and mixed solitary papillomas and in papillomatosis.

Malignant Tumours

Squamous Cell Carcinoma

Squamous cell carcinomas show the highest frequency of P53 mutations (50%–75%) of all histological types of lung carcinoma. P53 is a tumour suppressor gene with functions in G1 arrest and apoptosis in cells with cytotoxic stress. P53 immunoreactivity is fairly correlated with P53 missense mutation in the gene sequence. However, other types of P53 mutation, found in approximately 20% of cases, lead to absence of functional P53 protein and are not recognized by immunohistochemistry. An influence of P53 status on prognosis has not been demonstrated, except in the very early stages. P53 protein overexpression and, less commonly, mutations may precede invasion. Abnormal P53 accumulation is reported in 10%–50% of dysplasias. There is increasing frequency and intensity of P53 immunostaining with higher grade dysplasia and positivity can be seen in 60%–90% of squamous cell carcinoma in situ.

Loss of protein expression of the tumour suppressor gene Rb is detected in only 15% of NSCLC using immunohistochemistry, with the same frequency in squamous and adenocarcinoma. In NSCLC Rb is frequently inactivated through deregulation of its phosphorylation pathway. Both CdK-inhibitor inactivation and cyclin D1 overexpression contribute to this indirect Rb inactivation. The CdK-inhibitor P16INK4 is inactivated and its protein product lost in 65% of squamous cell carcinomas. Immunohistochemistry is a straightforward method to detect p16INK4 inactivation. Cyclin D1 overexpression secondary to amplification is observed in 45% of NSCLC. There is an inverse relation between Rb and P16, although about 30% of NSCLC display a Rb-positive/P16-positive phenotype. Cyclin D1 overexpression is directly related to the presence of Rb expression since only exceptional cases display cyclin D1 overexpression in the absence of Rb expression. However, 45% of cases display a Rb-positive/cyclin D1-negative phenotype.

Multiple allelic losses are observed in squamous cell carcinomas such as 3p (FHIT), 9p (P16), 17p (P53), 13q (Rb), 5q (APC MCC), 1q, 2q, 8q, at locations bearing tumour suppressor gene (indicated in parentheses). These tumour suppressor gene deletions, especially 3p, 9p- and 17p-, may precede invasion and be detected in histologically normal cells in smokers. *Ras* mutations are rare or absent in squamous cell carcinomas. Overexpression of epidermal growth factor receptor (EGF-r) has been detected in 80% of squamous cell carcinomas, but it is rarely mutated.

Small Cell Carcinoma and Other Neuroendocrine Lung Tumours

P53 and Rb tumour suppressor genes are frequently mutated in high-grade neuroendocrine lung tumours, including SCLC and LCNEC. P53 mutation and/or P53 protein accumulation are seen in 50%–80% of SCLC and LCNEC. Typical carcinoids have no P53 mutations and atypical carcinoids show P53 protein overexpression in 20%–40% of cases with uncommon mutations. Both SCLC and LCNEC share a high frequency of Rb loss of protein expression (80%–100%), detectable by immunohistochemistry. Loss of heterozygosity (LOH) at the 13q14 chromosomal locus of Rb is highly correlated with loss of protein expression in both LCNEC and SCLC. In contrast, the expression of P16INK4 is almost always maintained in Rb-negative SCLC and LCNEC. Typical carcinoids have retained Rb expression and have no

Rb mutation. Rb expression may be lost in up to 20% of atypical carcinoids. Most carcinoids show normal expression of P16INK4.

Immunohistochemistry for the anti-apoptotic gene *bcl2* is intensely expressed in 90% of SCLC and LCNEC in contrast with a low frequency of expression of the apoptotic gene, *bax*. The high grade SCLC and LCNEC display the same profile of genetic and molecular alterations of P53 and *bcl2/bax* ratio. These alterations are not seen in typical carcinoids and are present in only 10%–20% of atypical carcinoids. The *bcl2/bax* imbalance is clearly delineated in high-grade vs low-grade neuroendocrine lung tumours and it is predictive of prognosis in the overall spectrum of neuroendocrine lung tumours. LOH at 3p, 13q14 (Rb), 9p and 5q22 has been found in all neuroendocrine tumour types, with an increasing frequency from typical carcinoid to LCNEC and SCLC. There is no difference between LCNEC and SCLC.

The gradual increase of molecular abnormalities along the spectrum of neuroendocrine lung tumours strongly supports the grading concept of typical carcinoid as low-grade, atypical carcinoid as intermediate-grade and LCNEC and SCLC as high-grade neuroendocrine lung tumours. MEN1 gene mutations and loss of heterozygosity at the MEN1 gene locus, (11q13), have been recently demonstrated in 65% of sporadic atypical carcinoids and appear to be specific for this tumour type. MEN1 mutations have not been found in SCLC. *Ras* mutations are not characteristic of any subtype of neuroendocrine lung tumour.

Adenocarcinoma

K-*ras* mutations are primarily seen in adenocarcinoma. Most K-*ras* mutations affect codon 12. The frequency of K-*ras* mutations is much lower in non-smokers (5%) than in smokers (30%). There are conflicting data as to whether K-*ras* mutations correlate with a favourable or unfavourable prognosis. P53, Rb and P16 mutation and protein inactivation have the same frequency in adenocarcinomas as in squamous cell carcinomas. LOH has a different distribution in squamous cell carcinoma and adenocarcinoma. The differences in allelo-type and K-*ras* mutations in adenocarcinoma compared to other histological types strongly suggest differences in pathogenesis.

Large Cell Carcinoma and Adenosquamous Carcinoma

There is no characteristic molecular abnormality for either large cell carcinoma or adenosquamous carcinoma.

**Carcinoma with Pleomorphic,
Sarcomatoid or Sarcomatous Elements**

Only a few studies have investigated the molecular characteristics of these tumours. One study suggested that there are less frequent P53 mutations in pleomorphic carcinomas compared with adenocarcinomas or squamous cell carcinomas. The finding of identical P53 mutations in both the epithelial and spindle cell components of a small number of pleomorphic carcinomas, as well as in biphasic pulmonary blastomas and carcinosarcomas, supports a monoclonal histogenesis for these tumours. Another study demonstrated P53 gene mutations in 40% of biphasic blastomas by immunohistochemical and molecular analysis. No mutations were found in well-differentiated fetal adenocarcinomas. This molecular difference is one reason for separating biphasic pulmonary blastoma from well-differentiated fetal adenocarcinoma. It is better placed in the group of carcinomas with pleomorphic, sarcomatoid or sarcomatous elements.

Soft Tissue Tumours

For sarcomas arising in the lung, the same molecular markers as seen in their soft tissue counterparts may be demonstrated. Examples include the specific t(X; 18) chromosomal translocation for synovial sarcoma, the chromosomal translocation t(11;22)(p13;q12) typically seen in desmoplastic round cell tumour, and the t(11;22)(q24;q12) chromosomal translocation characteristic of Ewing sarcoma and primitive neuroectodermal tumour. Approximately half of fibrous tumours of pleura have cytogenetic abnormalities of the chromosome 19p.

Mesothelial Tumours

Cytogenetic studies have shown that approximately 60%–80% of malignant mesotheliomas have deletions in chromosomes 1p, 3p, 6q, 9p or 22q. Malignant mesotheliomas have a low frequency of P53 mutations, although P53 accumulation can be detected immunohisto-chemically in 70% of malignant mesotheliomas. This abnormal accumulation of P53 in malignant mesothelioma has several possible explanations including the formation of complexes with mdm2 protein with stabilization of wt P53 or binding of SV40 large T-antigen to P53 protein. It is likely that SV40 large T-antigen binds both P53 and Rb in malignant mesothelioma, inactivating both tumour suppressor genes. It is controversial whether SV40 contributes to the development of human malignant mesotheliomas.

Wilms tumour 1 susceptibility gene (WT1) product is selectively expressed in malignant mesothelioma. This overexpression has not yet been related to a specific mutation in the gene sequence. It has been proposed as an immunohistochemical marker for differentiation between mesothelioma and adenocarcinoma.

LOH could define a critical region in chromosome 1p22 commonly deleted in human malignant mesotheliomas: 74% of mesotheliomas tested showed a 1p deletion, most of them at the 1p21–22 region.

Miscellaneous Tumours

Pulmonary chondroid hamartomas have a specific genetic alteration, which is a 6p21 rearrangement that activates a high mobility group gene, HMGI (Y). This encodes a nuclear protein, with both chromatin-structural and gene-regulatory roles. HMGI (Y) rearrangement appears as the molecular basis for the majority of pulmonary hamartomas. A 12q14–15 rearrangement has also been shown in pulmonary chondroid hamartoma. These molecular abnormalities indicate that chondroid hamartomas are benign neoplasms rather than tumour-like lesions as previously classified in the 1981 WHO classification[8].

Monoclonality was recently shown for sclerosing hemangiomas using the human androgen X-chromosome-linked polymorphic marker and the phosphoglycerate kinase gene. Several inflammatory pseudotumours (inflammatory myofibroblastic tumours) have been shown to have clonal chromosomal abnormalities. In one case cytogenetics revealed a single clonal abnormality: t(1;2)(q21;p23) and del(4)(q27). This suggests that some of these are neoplastic.

---

[8] World Health Organization (1981) Histological typing of lung tumors, 2nd edn. WHO, Geneva

Histological Classification of Lung and Pleural Tumours

---

[1]Morphology code of the International Classification of Diseases for Oncology (ICD-O) and the Systematized Nomenclature of Medicine (SNOMED). Behaviour is coded /0 for benign tumours, /1 for low or uncertain malignant potential or borderline malignancy, /2 for in situ lesions and /3 for malignant tumours.
[2]The italicised numbers are provisional codes proposed for the third edition of ICD-O. They should, for the most part, be incorporated into the next edition of ICD-O, but they are subject to change.

1.3   *Malignant*

4   Miscellaneous Tumours

5   Lymphoproliferative Diseases

6   Secondary Tumours

7   Unclassified Tumours

8   Tumour-Like Lesions

Definitions and Explanatory Notes

1 Epithelial Tumours

1.1 Benign

1.1.1 Papillomas

1.1.1.1 Squamous cell papilloma

A papillary tumour consisting of delicate connective tissue fronds with a squamous epithelial surface. Non-keratinizing squamous epithelium may appear transitional.

1.1.1.1.1 Exophytic (Fig. 1)

1.1.1.1.2 Inverted (Figs. 2, 3)

Most papillomas are exophytic, but, rarely, inverted papillomas occur similar to those seen in the upper respiratory tract. Squamous papillomas may be multiple (papillomatosis) or solitary. The latter are seen more often in the bronchi of elderly smokers. Papillomatosis frequently presents in children (juvenile papillomatosis), but it can occur in adults. Solitary papillomas in adults may progress to papillomatosis. Human papilloma virus (HPV), usually types 6 or 11, can be demonstrated in some solitary or multiple squamous papillomas. Koilocytosis may be seen. Bronchial papillomatosis may progress to dysplasia, as well as in situ and invasive squamous cell carcinoma. HPV types 16, 18 and occasionally 11 are sometimes identified in squamous papillomas associated with carcinoma.

Bronchial papillomatosis usually occurs in the setting of laryngeal and tracheal papillomatosis, but isolated bronchial involvement may rarely occur. Papillomatosis can extend beyond the bronchus into the lung parenchyma, resulting in squamous cells filling adjacent alveoli or forming larger cystic lesions lined by non-keratinizing squamous epithelium.

1.1.1.2   Glandular papilloma *(Fig. 4)*

A papillary tumour lined by ciliated or non-ciliated columnar cells, with varying numbers of cuboidal cells and goblet cells.

These tumours are generally solitary and no malignant potential is recognized. These may be central (bronchial) or peripheral (bronchiolar).

1.1.1.3   Mixed squamous cell and glandular papilloma *(Fig. 5)*

A bronchial papilloma showing a mixture of squamous and glandular epithelium.

These papillomas are usually solitary, but they may be multifocal. The squamous epithelium in these papillomas is susceptible to dysplasia and progression to squamous carcinoma.

1.1.2   Adenomas

1.1.2.1   Alveolar adenoma *(Figs. 6, 7)*

A solitary nodule in the periphery of the lung consisting of a network of spaces lined by a simple low cuboidal epithelium. The stroma can range from thin, inconspicuous connective tissue to broad accumulations of spindle cells, sometimes with a myxoid matrix.

This tumour is liable to be mistaken for a lymphangioma, from which it differs histologically by the lining cells being more cuboidal than flattened. Ultrastructurally and immunohistochemically these lining cells are type II pneumocytes.

1.1.2.2   Papillary adenoma *(Figs. 8, 9)*

A circumscribed nodule consisting of a papillary growth of cuboidal to low-columnar epithelial cells lining the surface of a fibrovascular stroma.

The lesions are usually solitary peripheral parenchymal nodules. The cells are mostly type II cells interspersed with variable numbers of Clara cells as shown by electron microscopy and immunohistochemistry. Eosinophilic nuclear inclusions may be present. Oxyphilic cytoplasmic changes may be focal or diffuse.

1.1.2.3   Adenomas of salivary-gland type

1.1.2.3.1   Mucous gland adenoma (Fig. 10)

A tumour of the tracheobronchial seromucinous glands and ducts. Mucus-filled cysts, tubules, glands and papillary formations are lined by a spectrum of epithelium including tall columnar cells, flattened cuboidal cells, goblet cells, oncocytic cells and clear cells.

These tumours lack intermediate cells or a squamous component. If there is a suggestion of either of these, the possibility of a low-grade mucoepidermoid carcinoma (see Sect. 1.3.8.1) must be considered. The tumours present as a solitary, circumscribed endobronchial mass, often in children or young adults.

1.1.2.3.2   Pleomorphic adenoma

A tumour with both epithelial and connective tissue differentiation, consisting of glands intermingled with myoepithelial cells in a myxoid and chondroid stroma.

This tumour is identical to its counterpart in the salivary glands.

1.1.2.3.3   Others

The terms "monomorphic adenoma" and "myoepithelioma" are appropriate for the very rare benign tumours of the tracheobronchial glands, differentiating respectively along purely epithelial or myoepithelial cell lines, but examples of either are exceptionally rare.

1.1.2.4   Mucinous cystadenoma (Figs. 11, 12)

A localized cystic mass filled with mucin and surrounded by a fibrous wall lined by well-differentiated, columnar mucinous epithelium.

Separation from mucinous cystadenocarcinoma may be difficult. The benign lesion lacks the criteria of a mucinous adenocarcinoma, such as invasive growth into the surrounding lung (e.g. spread of mucin or mucinous epithelium into surrounding alveoli or lepidic growth, as seen in bronchioloalveolar carcinoma), and significant atypia and prominent pseudostratification. The mucinous epithelium may range from tall columnar to low cuboidal cells. Inflammation and fibrosis of the cyst wall tend to cause flattening or loss of the epithelium, in which case there may be a giant cell reaction to the mucin. In some cases, mild atypia may be present.

1.1.2.5   Others

Rare adenomas do not fall into the above categories.

1.2   Preinvasive lesions

Three types of preinvasive epithelial lesions are recognized: (1) squamous dysplasia and carcinoma in situ, (2) atypical adenomatous hyperplasia and (3) diffuse idiopathic pulmonary neuroendocrine cell hyperplasia (DIPNECH).

Preinvasive bronchial squamous lesions are subdivided into dysplasia and carcinoma in situ. The term preinvasive does not imply that progression to invasion will necessarily occur. These lesions represent a continuum of cytologic and histological changes that may show some overlap between defined categories. The criteria for the grades of dysplasia and for carcinoma in situ are summarized in Table 1 (p. 2 and 3). The morphologic continuum and infrequency of these lesions in biopsy specimens contribute to problems in reproducibility of diagnostic criteria, and the clinical significance of this grading system remains to be established. A variety of bronchial epithelial hyperplasias and metaplasias may occur that are not regarded as preneoplastic, including goblet cell hyperplasia, basal cell (reserve cell) hyperplasia, immature squamous metaplasia and squamous metaplasia. Carcinoma in situ refers to a preinvasive lesion that involves the entire thickness of the epithelium and shows the cellular and architectural features of carcinoma without penetration of the subepithelial basement membrane. Extension into submucosal glands does not constitute invasion provided the basement membrane is intact. Rarely, the bronchial mucosa may show *micropapillary change* that can make grading of dysplasia and separation from carcinoma in situ problematic due to distorted orientation of the epithelium. In the setting of inflammation, or following a biopsy or therapy, atypia should be assessed with restraint.

Dysplastic lesions of the bronchioloalveolar type are peripheral lesions, often situated in a peribronchiolar location that are generically designated atypical adenomatous hyperplasias.

Very rarely, carcinoid tumours arise in the setting of DIPNECH. Sometimes, this lesion is associated with multiple carcinoid tumourlets and/or peripheral carcinoid tumours. Neuroendocrine proliferations encompass a spectrum from neuroendocrine cell hyperplasia to tumourlets and carcinoid tumours (Table 2, p. 5), and arbitrary criteria are used to separate the lesions within this continuum (Table 2). Tumourlets represent micronodular neuroendocrine cell proliferations, usually extending beyond the bronchial/bronchiolar wall and forming aggregates of less than 0.5 cm in diameter (see Sect. 8.1). Arbitrarily, neuroendocrine proliferations measuring 0.5 cm or greater are called carcinoid tumours (see Sect. 1.3.7).

1.2.1   Squamous dysplasia/squamous cell carcinoma in situ
(Fig. 13)

Squamous dysplasia and carcinoma in situ resemble the same epithelial abnormalities in the upper aerodigestive tract and uterine cervix. Dysplastic changes may be mild, moderate or severe, but they fall short of the full thickness involvement that characterizes carcinoma in situ (see Table 1, p. 2 and 3). Koilocytotic changes are rarely seen in the bronchus. (*Other related term*: atypical squamous metaplasia.)

1.2.2   Atypical adenomatous hyperplasia (Figs. 14, 15)

A focal lesion, often 5 mm or less in diameter, in which the involved alveoli and respiratory bronchioles are lined by monotonous, slightly atypical cuboidal to low columnar epithelial cells with dense nuclear chromatin, inconspicuous nucleoli and scant cytoplasm.

These lesions resemble, but fall short of, criteria for bronchioloalveolar carcinoma, non-mucinous type. Alveolar septa are slightly thickened and may be infiltrated with lymphocytes. The degree of atypia varies from mild to severe and may overlap that seen in bronchioloalveolar carcinoma of Clara cell/type II pneumocyte type. Eosinophilic intranuclear inclusions may be found, but mitotic figures are rarely seen. Ultrastructurally, the epithelial cells resemble either type II pneumocytes or Clara cells. Some have used the term "bronchioloalveolar (cell) adenoma" for these lesions, but in the lung the term "adenoma" has historically been used for the group of entities discussed in Sect. 1.1.2 above, most of which are not "preinvasive". This entity has been defined primarily in the setting of resected lung cancer specimens, therefore little is known about the potential for progression to carcinoma. Several studies suggest that this risk is very low even with multicentric lesions. Grading of atypical adenomatous hyperplasia is not encouraged due to problems in reproducibility. (*Synonyms*: atypical alveolar cuboidal cell hyperplasia, alveolar epithelial hyperplasia, alveolar atypical hyperplasia, atypical alveolar hyperplasia, bronchioloalveolar adenoma and atypical bronchioloalveolar cell hyperplasia.)

1.2.3   Diffuse idiopathic pulmonary neuroendocrine cell hyperplasia (Figs. 16–18)

A proliferation of neuroendocrine cells confined to the bronchiolar epithelium. It consists of increased numbers of scattered single cells, small nodules (neuroendocrine bodies) or linear proliferations of neuroendocrine cells within the bronchiolar epithelium. While it is typically associated with obliterative bronchiolar fibrosis, underlying conditions causing interstitial or airway fibrosis or inflammation should be absent.

DIPNECH is a very rare clinicopathologic syndrome that is best documented in the setting of obstructive pulmonary function and lack of underlying interstitial lung disease as well as the characteristic histologic findings. Neuroendocrine cell hyperplasias are confined to the airway mucosa, without penetration through the basement membrane. Some neuroendocrine cell hyperplasias are associated with tumourlets. The neuroendocrine cells of tumourlets usually extend beyond the basement membrane and bronchiolar wall to form small nodules. While tumourlets are in this respect invasive, they are classified as "tumour-like lesions" (see Sect. 8.1) rather than neoplasms since they are incidental microscopic findings seen most often in a reactive setting associated with airway inflammation or interstitial fibrosis. Lymph node metastases from tumourlets are extremely rare.

Neuroendocrine cell hyperplasia is seen most often as a non-specific reaction, secondary to airway or interstitial inflammation and/or fibrosis. Therefore, most neuroendocrine cell hyperplasias probably do not represent a preneoplastic condition. Neuroendocrine cell hyperplasia is also found in the mucosa of bronchi or bronchioles adjacent to peripheral carcinoid tumours in up to 75% of cases. Whether these hyperplastic neuroendocrine cells represent a local reaction to the tumour or a localized preneoplastic condition is uncertain.

DIPNECH occurs in the absence of airway inflammation or diffuse interstitial fibrosis. A subset of these patients has multiple tumourlets and one or more peripheral carcinoid tumours. In this setting it appears that the neuroendocrine cell hyperplasia represents a preneoplastic lesion. Due to the rarity of these cases little is known concerning the percentage of patients who will develop carcinoid tumours, or how long it takes for the tumours to develop. The obstructive airway disease can be severe and require lung transplantation. Substances produced by the neuroendocrine cells may promote the airway fibrosis.

1.3   Malignant

1.3.1   Squamous cell carcinoma (Figs. 19–25)

A malignant epithelial tumour showing keratinization and/or intercellular bridges.

Keratinization may take the form of squamous pearls or individual cells with markedly eosinophilic dense cytoplasm. These features are prominent in well-differentiated tumours, but focal in poorly differentiated tumours. The presence of intracellular mucin in a few cells does not exclude tumours from this category. In situ squamous cell carcinoma may be seen in the adjacent airway mucosa.

In the past most squamous cell carcinomas arose centrally from the segmental or subsegmental bronchi. However, the incidence of squamous cell carcinoma of the peripheral lung is increasing. Some squamous cell carcinomas undergo cavitation.

Variants

1.3.1.1   Papillary (Figs. 22, 23)

1.3.1.2   Clear cell

1.3.1.3   Small cell (Fig. 24)

1.3.1.4   Basaloid (Fig. 25)

Squamous cell carcinomas can present as histological variants which include: *papillary, clear cell, small cell and basaloid* patterns. Rarely, these patterns are seen throughout the tumour, but more commonly they are focal. Some of the proximal tumours have an exophytic, *papillary* and endobronchial growth pattern. Even though invasive growth is not identified, *papillary* squamous cell carcinoma can be diagnosed if there is sufficient cytologic atypia. Small biopsy specimens that show very well differentiated papillary squamous epithelium should be interpreted with caution since separation of a *papillary* squamous carcinoma from a papilloma can be difficult. The pattern of verrucous carcinoma is very rare in the lung and is included under *papillary* squamous carcinoma. The *small cell* variant is a poorly differentiated squamous cell carcinoma with small tumour cells that retain morphologic characteristics of a non-small cell carcinoma and show focal squamous differentiation. This variant of squamous carcinoma must be distinguished from combined small cell carcinoma (see

Sect. 1.3.2.1) in which there is a mixture of squamous cell carcinoma and true small cell carcinoma. The small cell variant of squamous cell carcinoma lacks the characteristic nuclear features of small cell carcinoma, having coarse or vesicular chromatin, more prominent nucleoli, more cytoplasm and more distinct cell borders. Focal intercellular bridges may be seen. Squamous cell carcinomas with prominent peripheral palisading of nuclei at the edge of tumour cell nests are called the *basaloid* variant of squamous cell carcinoma. Poorly differentiated carcinomas with an extensive basaloid pattern but lacking squamous differentiation are called basaloid carcinoma and are regarded as a variant of large cell carcinoma (see Sect. 1.3.4.2). The issue of pleomorphic carcinoma (spindle cell or sarcomatoid carcinoma) is addressed below (see Sect. 1.3.6.1). Rare non-keratinizing squamous cell carcinomas resemble a transitional cell carcinoma.

Squamous cell carcinomas are graded as well-differentiated if they show extensive keratinization, intercellular bridges or pearl formation. They are moderately differentiated if these features are easily seen but not extensive. Poorly differentiated squamous cell carcinomas have only focal morphologic features of squamous differentiation; the remaining component usually has the pattern of a large cell carcinoma. Mitotic activity is higher in poorly differentiated tumours.

1.3.2   Small cell carcinoma (Figs. 26–32)

A malignant epithelial tumour consisting of small cells with scant cytoplasm, ill-defined cell borders, finely granular nuclear chromatin and absent or inconspicuous nucleoli. The cells are round, oval and spindle-shaped and nuclear molding is prominent. The mitotic count is high.

Variant

1.3.2.1   Combined small cell carcinoma (Figs. 29–32)

A small cell carcinoma combined with an additional component that consists of any of the histological types of non-small cell carcinoma, usually adenocarcinoma, squamous cell carcinoma or large cell carcinoma, but less commonly spindle cell or giant cell carcinoma. The type of non-small cell carcinoma should be specified, e.g. combined small cell and adenocarcinoma.

In the 1981 classification three subtypes of small cell carcinoma were proposed: (1) oat cell carcinoma, (2) small cell carcinoma, intermediate cell type, and (3) combined oat cell carcinoma[1]. Problems that were subsequently recognized included difficulties in reproducibility and lack of demonstrable clinical significance. In 1988, the International Association for the Study of Lung Cancer (IASLC) pathology panel proposed the following three subtypes: (1) *small cell carcinoma*, (2) *mixed small cell/large cell carcinoma*, and (3) *combined small cell carcinoma*. It was also recommended that the terms "oat cell carcinoma" and "intermediate cell type" be dropped and that all tumours with pure histology simply be called *small cell carcinoma*. The category of *mixed small cell/large cell carcinoma* was defined as a tumour with components of both small cell and large cell carcinoma, but subsequent studies did not clearly confirm clinical significance or interobserver reproducibility for this category. The category of *combined small cell carcinoma* included cases with a mixture of small cell and squamous cell carcinoma or adenocarcinoma. We propose that the term "small cell carcinoma" alone be used for tumours of pure histology without a non-small cell component. A single variant of small cell carcinoma is recognized: *combined small cell carcinoma* in which there is a mixture of small cell carcinoma and *any other* non-small cell component including large cell neuroendocrine carcinoma (LCNEC). The histological type of the non-small cell carcinoma component should be noted in the diagnosis. If the tumour has a component of heterologous sarcomatous elements then it is a combined small cell carcinoma and sarcoma and is classified primarily as a variant of small cell carcinoma rather than as a carcinosarcoma.

Small cell carcinoma occurs both in major bronchi and in the periphery of the lung. It destroys and may undermine, but rarely replaces the bronchial epithelium. Small cell carcinoma is not known to have a preinvasive phase of carcinoma in situ. Squamous dysplasia and carcinoma in situ may be seen in adjacent bronchial or bronchiolar epithelium, but the presence of these lesions is more often associated with a poorly differentiated squamous cell carcinoma, and the diagnosis of small cell carcinoma should be made with caution in such a setting.

In open biopsy specimens it is evident that small cell carcinomas have a high mitotic rate that averages 60–70 per 2 mm^2 (ten high-

---

[1]World Health Organization (1981) Histological typing of lung tumors,
2nd edn. WHO, Geneva

power fields), ranging up to over 200 per 2 mm² (ten high-power fields) (Table 3, p. 8). The degree of mitotic activity is usually also appreciated on a well-preserved open biopsy specimen, but it may be more difficult to see mitoses in small, crushed bronchoscopic biopsies. Assessing the high mitotic rate is important in separating small cell carcinomas from typical and atypical carcinoids.

There is no absolute size for the tumour cells of small cell carcinoma, but in general the tumour cells should be less than the size of three small resting lymphocytes. Cell size is greater in larger, well-fixed specimens and frozen sections.

Necrosis is common and often extensive, although it may not be seen in a small bronchoscopic or needle biopsy. Basophilic staining of vascular walls due to encrustation by DNA from necrotic tumour cells (the Azzopardi effect) is frequent in areas of necrosis, but is not specific for small cell carcinoma.

Crush artifact may preclude a definite diagnosis since this artifact and DNA encrustation may be seen in other highly cellular tumours and in inflammatory conditions.

Small cell carcinoma is a light microscopic diagnosis and does not require a demonstration of neuroendocrine differentiation by electron microscopy or immunohistochemistry. Electron microscopy shows neuroendocrine granules of approximately 100 nm in diameter in at least two thirds of cases. Immunohistochemistry can be negative for neuroendocrine markers such as chromogranin, synaptophysin and Leu-7 in about 25% of cases.

Grading is inappropriate since all small cell carcinomas are high grade.

1.3.3   Adenocarcinoma

A malignant epithelial tumour with glandular differentiation or mucin production by the tumour cells showing acinar (Fig. 33), papillary (Fig. 34), bronchioloalveolar (Figs. 35–39), or solid with mucin formation (Fig. 40) growth patterns or a mixture of these patterns (Figs. 41, 42).

Adenocarcinoma is increasing in frequency and accounts for almost half of lung cancers in some countries. It is associated with cigarette smoking, but less strongly than the other major histological types. Rare adenocarcinomas with a pseudomesotheliomatous growth pattern cause a rind-like thickening of the pleura like a malignant mesothelioma.

Some primary adenocarcinomas of the lung resemble carcinomas of the breast and salivary gland, while others, particularly those of signet-ring cell type, may be very similar to those originating in the gastrointestinal tract. However, most adenocarcinomas of the lung differentiate toward the peripheral airway Clara cells and type II pneumocytes.

Immunohistochemical evaluation for surfactant proteins, thyroid transcription factor-1, prostate-specific antigen, prostatic acid phosphatase, keratin 7 vs keratin 20, estrogen or progesterone receptors and villin can help distinguish between primary pulmonary adenocarcinomas and metastatic adenocarcinomas from other organs.

Individual adenocarcinomas frequently display mixed histology, combining bronchioloalveolar, papillary, acinar, tubular and solid growth patterns. Therefore, it is difficult to apply adenocarcinoma subtypes of the 1981 classification. Small adenocarcinomas (i.e. less than 2 cm in diameter) more often consist of a single cell type and display a uniform histological pattern.

In most adenocarcinomas where prominent mucin is present, further histological sampling will reveal an acinar or papillary growth pattern. The tumour cells are polygonal with large vesicular nuclei, prominent nucleoli and moderately abundant cytoplasm. Adenocarcinoma composed of solid nests with many mucin-containing tumour cells and a few to occasional acini is called poorly differentiated acinar adenocarcinoma.

In contrast with bronchioloalveolar carcinoma, the other histological subtypes of adenocarcinoma (acinar, papillary, solid and mixed) can arise anywhere from bronchi to alveoli and thus may grow as an endobronchial or a peripheral lung mass.

Histological grading of adenocarcinomas by degree of differentiation may be carried out by applying conventional histological criteria to architectural patterns and cytologic features. Tumours with a solid component will be poorly differentiated.

The mixed subtype is the most frequent adenocarcinoma encountered in routine practice. There is usually a mixture of acinar, papillary, solid with mucin formation and bronchioloalveolar patterns, but any of these may be seen in pure form.

Adenocarcinomas are divided according to the following sections.

1.3.3.1   Acinar (Fig. 33)

An adenocarcinoma with acini and tubules composed frequently of mucin producing cells resembling bronchial gland or bronchial lining epithelial cells.

1.3.3.2   Papillary (Fig. 34)

An adenocarcinoma with a predominance of papillary structures that replaces the underlying alveolar architecture.

There are two types of papillary structures: one consists of cuboidal to low columnar, non-mucinous (Clara cells/type II pneumocytes) replacing alveolar lining cells and displaying complicated secondary and tertiary papillary branches; the other consists of tall columnar or cuboidal cells with or without mucin production growing with their own fibrovascular stroma and invading lung parenchyma.

1.3.3.3   Bronchioloalveolar carcinoma (Figs. 35–39)

An adenocarcinoma with a pure bronchioloalveolar growth pattern and no evidence of stromal, vascular or pleural invasion.

There may be some increase in thickness of alveolar septa and a central or subpleural area of alveolar collapse with increased elastic fibers. Since this definition requires exclusion of an invasive component, this tumour cannot be diagnosed on small biopsy specimens. A bronchioloalveolar pattern may be recognized in a small biopsy specimen, but the final diagnosis requires thorough histological sampling of a resected specimen. In such cases the term "adenocarcinoma, possible bronchioloalveolar carcinoma" is appropriate with an explanatory comment. If an invasive component is identified then the tumour is classified as "adenocarcinoma mixed bronchioloalveolar (and acinar or papillary, if present) subtype" (see Sect. 1.3.3.5, Figs. 40, 41) rather than pure bronchioloalveolar carcinoma (see Sect. 1.3.3.3).

1.3.3.3.1   Non-mucinous (Figs. 35–37)

A non-mucinous adenocarcinoma with Clara cells and/or type II pneumocytes growing along alveolar walls and without stromal invasion.

Clara cells are columnar or peg-shaped with cytoplasmic snouts and eosinophilic cytoplasm. Some nuclei are located in the apical cytoplasm. Diastase-predigested periodic acid–Schiff-positive cytoplasmic granules may be present. The degree of cell atypia varies, as do nuclear and nucleolar size. Type II cells are cuboidal or dome-shaped with fine cytoplasmic vesicles, or even clear foamy cytoplasm. Intranuclear eosinophilic inclusions with a clear halo may be noted with either cell type. It is not necessary to specifically identify these cell types for routine diagnosis. Aerogenous spread is rarely seen.

This histological subtype of bronchioloalveolar carcinoma is reasonably distinctive, suggesting a lung primary in most instances.

Non-mucinous bronchioloalveolar carcinomas often consist of a peripheral lung nodule showing recognizable alveolar spaces and blurred borders on cut section. Indentation of the pleura associated with subpleural or central anthracotic and fibrotic foci are seen in some bronchioloalveolar carcinomas without stromal invasion, and in the large majority of adenocarcinomas with a predominantly bronchioloalveolar pattern.

Bronchioloalveolar carcinomas of this type are often associated with central alveolar collapse (fibrosis) and have been interpreted erroneously as scar cancers. Stromal invasion is suggested by tumour cells arranged in acinic, papillotubular structures or solid nests of non-mucinous cells (Clara cell/type II pneumocytes) in a fibroblastic stroma, often accompanied by collagenization, as well as cytologic atypia and mucin production. Invasive growth includes penetration into the pleura, as well as invasion of lymphatics or vessels or metastases. Elastic stains may highlight pleural and vascular invasion.

Papillary growth with complicated secondary and tertiary branches lined by Clara cells or type II pneumocytes is classified as papillary adenocarcinoma (see Sect. 1.3.3.2) since overt invasive growth is very often noted in other parts of the tumour.

Compared with atypical adenomatous hyperplasia (see Sect. 1.2.2), bronchioloalveolar carcinoma shows increased cytologic atypia, more columnar cells and greater crowding of cells and it is typically greater than 5 mm (usually at least 1 cm) in size.

Electron microscopy confirms features of Clara cells or type II pneumocytes or a combination of two cell types. Recent studies suggest a close association with, or development from, atypical adenomatous hyperplasia (see Sect. 1.2.2).

1.3.3.3.2   Mucinous (Figs. 38, 39)

A mucinous adenocarcinoma composed of tall columnar cells, with varying amounts of cytoplasmic mucin, which typically displace the nucleus to the base of the cell, growing along alveolar walls and without stromal invasion.

Alveolar spaces are frequently distended with mucin. Nuclear atypia is mild, the nuclei varying from small and densely stained to medium-sized with small nucleoli.

This tumour tends to spread aerogenously, forming satellite tumours in the lungs. The tumour may present as a solitary nodule, as multiple nodules or an entire lobe may be consolidated by tumour, resembling lobar pneumonia (diffuse pneumonic variant). This pattern of bronchioloalveolar carcinoma may be mimicked by secondary adenocarcinoma metastatic to the lung. A precursor lesion, analogous to atypical adenomatous hyperplasia for non-mucinous bronchioloalveolar carcinoma, has not been identified.

1.3.3.3.3   Mixed mucinous and non-mucinous or indeterminate cell type

An adenocarcinoma with a mixture of mucinous and non-mucinous cells or one in which it is not possible to distinguish the two cell types. The tumour grows along alveolar walls without stromal invasion.

Mixed mucinous and non-mucinous bronchioloalveolar carcinomas are very rare.

1.3.3.4   Solid adenocarcinoma with mucin *(Fig. 40)*

An adenocarcinoma lacking acini, tubules and papillae, but with frequent mucin-containing tumour cells (five or more mucin-positive cells in at least two high-power fields).

Histochemical stains for mucin such as mucicarmine or periodic acid–Schiff with diastase digestion can be helpful in distinguishing these tumours from large cell carcinoma. Rare mucin droplets can be seen in squamous cell carcinomas and large cell carcinomas. If the presence of mucin is suspected on review of hematoxylin and eosin-stained sections, then mucin stains are appropriate and a considerable amount of mucin, as specified above, rather than focal mucin droplets, should be required for classification in this category. Mucin stains do not need to be performed on every squamous cell carcinoma or large cell carcinoma.

1.3.3.5   Adenocarcinoma with mixed subtypes

The majority of adenocarcinomas show a mixture of the above histological subtypes. These tumours are called "adenocarcinomas" and the various patterns identified may be addressed in a comment. For example, adenocarcinomas with a prominent bronchioloalveolar pattern that have an invasive component should be called adenocarcinoma mixed bronchioloalveolar and acinar (or whatever other patterns on identified) (Figs. 41, 42).

1.3.3.6   *Variants*

1.3.3.6.1   Well-differentiated fetal adenocarcinoma (Fig. 43)

1.3.3.6.2   Mucinous ("colloid") adenocarcinoma (Figs. 44, 45)

1.3.3.6.3   Mucinous cystadenocarcinoma

1.3.3.6.4   Signet-ring adenocarcinoma (Fig. 46)

1.3.3.6.5   Clear cell adenocarcinoma

Adenocarcinomas can rarely show a pattern resembling fetal lung tubules (*well-differentiated fetal adenocarcinoma*). The epithelial component has a distinctive appearance consisting of glandular elements composed of tubules of glycogen-rich, non-ciliated cells that resemble fetal lung tubules. Subnuclear and supranuclear glycogen vacuoles give the tumour an endometrioid appearance. Rounded morules of polygonal cells with abundant eosinophilic and finely granular cytoplasm are common. The tumours may have a predominant clear cell pattern. In rare cases a mixture of well-differentiated fetal adenocarcinoma and other common subtypes of adenocarcinoma may be encountered. The well-differentiated fetal adenocarcinoma pattern may be seen as the epithelial component of *pulmonary blastomas* that have a biphasic pattern (see Sect. 1.3.6.3). Therefore, on a small biopsy specimen, one cannot exclude the possibility of a biphasic *pulmonary blastoma* if the pattern of *well-differentiated fetal adenocarcinoma* is identified. The term pulmonary blastoma been used for both *well-differentiated fetal adenocarcinoma* and biphasic *pulmonary blastoma*. These are distinct from pleuropulmonary blastoma (see Sect. 2.3). However, *well-differentiated fetal adenocarcinoma* is now included as a histological variant of adenocarcinoma and distinguished from biphasic *pulmonary blastoma* since the former has a much better prognosis and lacks the P53 mutations seen in the latter. (*Synonyms*: pulmonary blastoma, epithelial type and pulmonary endodermal tumour resembling fetal lung.)

Several other histological variants of adenocarcinoma may be encountered either as a focal pattern associated with one of the other major subtypes or rarely as a pure histological pattern. *Mucinous (colloid) adenocarcinoma* is similar to the tumour of the same name in the gastrointestinal tract. Tumour cells float in pools of mucin which often distend alveoli. *Mucinous cystadenocarcinoma* is a cystic adenocarcinoma with copious mucin production. It may resemble tumours of the same name in the ovary, breast and pancreas. Adenocarcinomas may also contain *signet-ring cells* and *clear cell* change.

Adenocarcinoma with spindle cell and/or giant cell features is classified under *pleomorphic carcinoma* (see Sect. 1.3.6.1).

1.3.4   Large cell carcinoma *(Fig. 47)*

An undifferentiated malignant epithelial tumour that lacks the cytologic features of small cell carcinoma and glandular or squamous differentiation. The cells typically have large nuclei, prominent nucleoli and a moderate amount of cytoplasm.

Large cell carcinoma is a diagnosis of exclusion made after ruling out the presence of a component of squamous cell carcinoma, adenocarcinoma or small cell carcinoma. Ultrastructurally, however, minimal glandular or squamous differentiation is common. If abundant mucin-producing cells can be demonstrated by mucin stains such as mucicarmine or periodic acid–Schiff with diastase digestion, the tumour is classified as solid adenocarcinoma with mucin formation. In most cases, the mucin production can be seen by routine light microscopy so mucin stains do not need to be performed on every large cell carcinoma unless intracytoplasmic or intercellular mucin is suspected. A few mucin-positive cells may be found in large cell carcinomas and squamous cell carcinomas.

Variants

1.3.4.1   Large cell neuroendocrine carcinoma (Figs. 48–50)

A large cell carcinoma showing histological features such as organoid nesting, trabecular, rosette-like and palisading patterns that suggest neuroendocrine differentiation and in which the latter can be confirmed by immunohistochemistry or electron microscopy.

The tumour cells are generally large, with moderate to abundant cytoplasm, and the nuclear chromatin ranges from vesicular to finely granular. Nucleoli are frequent and often prominent and their presence facilitates separation from small cell carcinoma. However, some tumours without nucleoli fulfill the criteria for a non-small cell carcinoma because of other morphologic features such as large cell size and abundance of cytoplasm. Mitotic counts are typically 11 or more per 2 mm^2 (ten high-power fields) area of viable tumour, (see Introduction, The Spectrum of Neuroendocrine Tumours), averaging 75 per 2 mm^2 area. Large zones of necrosis are common. The term *large cell carcinoma with neuroendocrine morphology* is used for tumors where the neuroendocrine markers are negative (see p. 12).

1.3.4.1.1   Combined large cell neuroendocrine carcinoma (Fig. 51)

A large cell neuroendocrine carcinoma with components of adeno-carcinoma, squamous cell carcinoma, giant cell carcinoma and/or spindle cell carcinoma.

Like small cell carcinoma, a small percentage of large cell neuroendocrine carcinomas are histologically heterogeneous. In view of the many shared clinical, epidemiologic, survival and neuroendocrine properties between large cell neuroendocrine carcinoma and small cell carcinoma, we have arbitrarily chosen to classify these tumours as combined large cell carcinoma until future studies better define their biological behaviour. Combinations with small cell carcinoma also occur, but such tumours are classified as combined variants of small cell carcinoma (see Sect. 1.3.2.1).

1.3.4.2   Basaloid carcinoma *(Figs. 52, 53)*

A large cell carcinoma with a basaloid appearance, including lobular, trabecular or palisading growth patterns, consisting of relatively small monomorphic cuboidal to fusiform cells with moderately hyperchromatic nuclei, finely granular chromatin, absent or only focal nucleoli, scant cytoplasm and a high mitotic rate. Neither intercellular bridges nor individual cell keratinization are present.

Comedo-type necrosis is common. Rosettes are seen in about one third of cases. Immunohistochemical stains for neuroendocrine markers are negative and no neurosecretory granules are seen by electron microscopy. About half of the tumours with this *histological* pattern are pure basaloid carcinomas and these are classified as a subtype of large cell carcinoma. The remaining cases have a minor (less than 50%) component of squamous cell carcinoma or adenocarcinoma, and are classified as squamous cell carcinoma (*basaloid variant*) or adenocarcinoma, respectively. A high percentage of cases (50%) have associated carcinoma in situ. Most of these tumours develop in proximal bronchi and they frequently have an endobronchial component. Patients seem to have a significantly shorter survival than those with poorly differentiated squamous cell carcinomas.

1.3.4.3   Lymphoepithelioma-like carcinoma *(Fig. 54)*

A large cell carcinoma histologically similar to nasopharyngeal lymphoepithelial carcinoma with nests of large malignant cells in a lymphoid-rich stroma.

Lymphoepithelioma-like carcinoma of the lung is very rare in Western countries, but not in Southeast Asia where it is frequently associated with Epstein-Barr virus.

1.3.4.4   Clear cell carcinoma (Fig. 55)

A large cell carcinoma with pure clear cell features.

Large polygonal tumour cells with water-clear or foamy cytoplasm characterize these tumours. Tumour cells may or may not contain glycogen. Clear cell carcinoma of the lung resembles metastatic clear cell carcinomas arising in organs such as the kidney, thyroid and salivary gland. If squamous or glandular differentiation is seen, the tumours are classified as clear cell variants of squamous cell or adenocarcinoma, respectively.

1.3.4.5   Large cell carcinoma with rhabdoid phenotype (Fig. 56)

A large cell carcinoma with cells showing prominent eosinophilic cytoplasmic globules.

The cytoplasmic globules consist of intermediate filaments, which may be positive for vimentin and cytokeratin. Lung carcinomas may have focal or extensive zones demonstrating a *rhabdoid phenotype*. However, the rhabdoid phenotype usually occurs in a poorly differentiated component of the tumour with the morphology of large cell carcinoma. Pure large cell carcinomas with a rhabdoid phenotype are very rare.

1.3.5   Adenosquamous carcinoma (Fig. 57)

A carcinoma showing components of both squamous cell carcinoma and adenocarcinoma with each comprising at least 10% of the whole tumour.

As there is a continuum of histological heterogeneity with both squamous cell and adenocarcinoma, the criteria of 10% for each component is arbitrary. Since some squamous cell carcinomas show focal mucin on histochemical stains the adenocarcinoma component is more easily defined if it shows an acinar, papillary or bronchioloalveolar pattern. The diagnosis of adenosquamous carcinoma is difficult if the adenocarcinoma component is confined to the pattern of solid adenocarcinoma with mucin formation.

1.3.6   Carcinomas with pleomorphic, sarcomatoid or sarcomatous elements

A group of poorly differentiated non-small cell carcinomas that contain a component of sarcoma or sarcoma-like elements.

These include tumours described under a variety of terms, including pleomorphic carcinoma, sarcomatoid carcinoma (monophasic and biphasic), spindle cell carcinoma, giant cell carcinoma, carcinosarcoma and blastoma, that may represent a continuum of epithelial and mesenchymal differentiation. Any small cell carcinoma with a component consisting of sarcoma-like features is classified as *combined small cell carcinoma* (see Sect. 1.3.2.1).

1.3.6.1   Carcinomas with spindle and/or giant cells

A poorly differentiated non-small cell carcinoma that contains spindle cells, giant cells or a mixture of these cell types.

1.3.6.1.1   Pleomorphic carcinoma (Figs. 58–61)

A poorly differentiated non-small cell carcinoma, namely squamous cell carcinoma, adenocarcinoma or large cell carcinoma containing spindle cells and/or giant cells or, a carcinoma consisting only of spindle cells and giant cells.

When a component of adenocarcinoma or squamous cell carcinoma is present in a pleomorphic carcinoma, it should be documented. Foci of large cell carcinoma are common in these tumours, but do not need to be specifically mentioned. The spindle cell and/or giant cell component should comprise at least 10% of the tumour. If a component of small cell carcinoma is found, the tumour is classified as a *combined small cell carcinoma* (see Sect. 1.3.2.2). Immunohistochemistry for epithelial markers such as keratin or epithelial membrane antigen can be useful to confirm carcinomatous differentiation in the spindle cell component, but even if the epithelial markers are negative these tumours are classified as pleomorphic carcinomas. Heterologous elements are required for the diagnosis of carcinosarcoma.

1.3.6.1.2   Spindle cell carcinoma

A carcinoma consisting only of spindle-shaped tumour cells.

The pure form of spindle cell carcinoma is very rare. Since it represents a histological continuum with pleomorphic carcinoma and shares the same aggressive behaviour it is classified in this general group of tumours. If the spindle cell component is combined with a component of squamous cell carcinoma, adenocarcinoma, giant cell carcinoma or large cell carcinoma, the tumour should be classified as *pleomorphic carcinoma* (see Sect. 1.3.6.1.1). Spindle cell carcinoma displays a sarcoma-like growth pattern, often exhibiting marked cellular pleomorphism and abnormal mitoses. It is frequently admixed with non-neoplastic connective tissue elements and may be combined with giant cell carcinoma, in which case the tumour is classified as pleomorphic carcinoma. Immunohistochemistry for epithelial markers may be useful to confirm epithelial differentiation. If keratin stains are negative separation from sarcoma is difficult.

1.3.6.1.3   Giant cell carcinoma (Figs. 62, 63)

A large cell carcinoma consisting only of highly pleomorphic multi- and/or mononucleated tumour giant cells.

Pure giant cell carcinoma is very rare. More often the pattern of giant cell carcinoma is associated with a spindle or large polygonal cell component, or a differentiated component such as adenocarcinoma in which case it is classified as *pleomorphic carcinoma* (see Sect. 1.3.6.1.1). Giant cell carcinoma consists of multi- or mononucleated, large, polygonal cells, often dyscohesive, with hyperchromatic, coarsely granular chromatin and distinct nucleoli. There is often infiltration or emperipolesis by polymorphonuclear leukocytes or lymphocytes. Giant cell carcinomas should be distinguished from the osteoclast-like giant cell inflammatory response that can occurs in malignant fibrous histiocytomas as well as the sarcomatoid component of pleomorphic carcinomas.

1.3.6.2   Carcinosarcoma (Figs. 64, 65)

A malignant tumour having a mixture of carcinoma and sarcoma containing heterologous elements such as malignant cartilage, bone or skeletal muscle. A similar tumour without heterologous elements is classified as pleomorphic carcinoma.

This separation is arbitrary, but intended to foster uniform classification.

1.3.6.3   Pulmonary blastoma (Figs. 66–68)

A biphasic tumour containing a primitive epithelial component that may resemble well-differentiated fetal adenocarcinoma and a primitive mesenchymal stroma, which occasionally has foci of osteosarcoma, chondrosarcoma or rhabdomyosarcoma.

The epithelial component has a distinctive primitive appearance, often resembling well-differentiated fetal adenocarcinoma (see Sect. 1.3.3.6.1). Squamoid morules are uncommon in biphasic tumours. The classic pulmonary blastoma presents mainly in adults, whereas pleuropulmonary blastoma (see Sect. 2.3) occurs almost exclusively in children of 6 years old or less at diagnosis.

1.3.6.4   Others

In rare cases there may be unusual tumours that are difficult to classi-fy that best fit into this category. Rare mixtures of carcinosarcoma and blastoma or blastoma and conventional adenocarcinoma may occur.

1.3.7   Carcinoid tumour (Figs. 69–74)

A tumour that is characterized by growth patterns such as organoid, trabecular, insular, palisading, ribbon or rosette-like arrangements which suggest neuroendocrine differentiation. The tumour cells have uniform cytologic features with moderate eosinophilic, finely granu-lar cytoplasm and nuclei with a finely granular chromatin pattern. Nucleoli may be present but are more frequent in atypical carcinoids.

In addition to the common trabecular, palisading, organoid or insu-lar patterns, carcinoids can have papillary, sclerosing, follicular and glandular features. Focal spindle cell and oxyphilic features are com-mon in carcinoids, but less often comprise the dominant histological pattern. Unusual cytologic features include mucin and melanin pro-duction and prominent nuclear convolutions. Stromal changes includ-ing bone, cartilage, dense fibrosis and amyloid can be seen. These tumours may be accompanied by neuroendocrine cell hyperplasia in the airway epithelium, sometimes associated with airway fibrosis. This is seen most often in association with peripheral carcinoids. In very rare cases the underlying condition of diffuse idiopathic neuroen-docrine cell hyperplasia is found, often with multiple tumourlets and sometimes with multiple carcinoid tumours.

1.3.7.1   Typical carcinoid *(Figs. 69–71)*

A carcinoid tumour with fewer than two mitoses per 2 mm² of viable tumour (ten high-power fields) and lacking necrosis. Some of these tumours show cytologic atypia, increased cellularity and lymphatic invasion.

1.3.7.2   Atypical carcinoid *(Figs. 73, 74)*

A carcinoid tumour with between two and ten mitoses per 2 mm² (ten high-power fields) and/or with foci of necrosis.

The necrosis is usually punctate. Other criteria, which are more sub-jective include cytologic atypia, lymphatic invasion, nucleoli, increased cellularity and disorganized architecture.

The number of mitoses is the most important criterion to separate atypical from typical carcinoids. On small biopsy specimens this may not be possible.

1.3.8   Carcinomas of salivary-gland type

These tumours are described in more detail in the WHO *Histological Classification of Tumours of the Salivary Gland*[2]. Some adenocarcinomas of the lung are probably of bronchial gland origin but are included under the heading of acinar adenocarcinoma (see Sect. 1.3.3.1) because they lack features that distinguish them as carcinomas of salivary-gland type.

1.3.8.1   Mucoepidermoid carcinoma (Fig. 75)

A malignant epithelial tumour characterized by the presence of squamoid cells, mucin-secreting cells and cells of intermediate type. It is histologically identical to the salivary gland tumour of the same name.

Mucoepidermoid carcinomas usually arise from segmental and subsegmental bronchi. Low-grade tumours may have prominent cystic change. Intermediate and/or squamoid cells may be focal, but their presence enables the distinction from mucous gland adenomas or mucin-producing adenocarcinomas. Clear cells and oxyphilic cells may be seen. Prominent stromal hyalinization and rarely chronic inflammation can be present.

Mucoepidermoid carcinoma of high-grade malignancy is differentiated from adenosquamous carcinoma (see Sect. 1.3.5) by a variety of features, including the characteristic admixture of mucin-containing cells and squamoid cells, a central endobronchial location, transition areas from classical low-grade mucoepidermoid carcinoma and lack of keratinization, squamous pearl formation or in situ squamous cell carcinoma.

1.3.8.2   Adenoid cystic carcinoma (Fig. 76)

A malignant epithelial tumour having a characteristic cribriform appearance, histologically identical to the salivary gland variety.

---

[2]World Health Organization (1991) Histological typing of salivary gland tumors, 2nd edn. Springer-Verlag, Berlin Heidelberg New York

This tumour should be differentiated from mucin-producing acinar adenocarcinoma with a cribriform pattern. Adenoid cystic carcinomas of the lower respiratory tract usually arise in the trachea and large bronchi.

1.3.8.3   *Others*

Other rare malignant salivary-gland type tumours, including acinic cell carcinoma, epimyoepithelial carcinoma and malignant mixed tumours, can arise from bronchial glands.

1.3.9   Unclassified carcinoma

A malignant epithelial neoplasm that cannot be placed into one of the above categories.

Some lung carcinomas remain unclassified. They usually fall into the "non-small cell carcinoma" category or are cases where small biopsy or cytology specimens preclude definitive histological typing.

2   Soft Tissue Tumours

A variety of soft tissue tumours arise in the lungs or pleura. Those that are benign include lipoma, localized fibrous tumour (fibroma, fibrous mesothelioma), chondroma, neurofibroma, neurilemoma, lymphangioma, hemangioma, leiomyoma, myxoma, granular cell tumour, glomus tumour and meningioma. Among the malignant tumours are fibrosarcoma, neurogenic sarcoma, angiosarcoma, lymphangiosarcoma, leiomyosarcoma, malignant fibrous histiocytoma, hemangiopericytoma, Kaposi sarcoma, chondrosarcoma, osteosarcoma, liposarcoma, rhabdomyosarcoma, alveolar soft part sarcoma, synovial sarcoma, pleuropulmonary blastoma, primitive neuroectodermal tumour and desmoplastic round cell tumour. These tumours are defined and classified according to the World Health Organization *Histological Typing of Soft Tissue Tumours*[3]. Several varieties of soft tissue tumours merit mention here.

---

[3]World Health Organization (1994) Histologic typing of soft tissue tumors, 2nd edn. Springer-Verlag, Berlin Heidelberg New York

2.1   Localized fibrous tumour (Figs. 77–80)

A tumour consisting of spindled fibroblastic cells arranged haphazardly around an elaborate, sometimes pericytoma-like, vasculature; hyalinization is a common feature.

Previously called "benign mesothelioma" or "benign fibrous mesothelioma" in the pleura and "fibroma" in the lung, localized fibrous tumours are now recognized as soft tissue tumours with a propensity to occur in the pleura and, less commonly, in the lung, as well as other sites. They are commonly attached to the visceral pleura by a pedicle. In the lung, they may be subpleural, lie adjacent to a fissure or be intraparenchymal in location.

Localized fibrous tumours are benign (Figs. 77, 78) or malignant, although this distinction may be difficult (Figs. 79, 80). They are usually solitary, but can present with more than one nodule. Grossly, benign tumours are whorled and fibrous-appearing on cut section, whereas malignant tumours are more fleshy and may show haemorrhage and necrosis. Sessile pleural tumours may be difficult to excise in their entirety, in which case recurrence is likely whether they are microscopically benign or malignant. Tumours on a pedicle are more easily resected and less apt to recur. Recurrences following resection tend to be in the form of multiple discrete nodules. Malignant localized fibrous tumours show pleomorphism, mitotic activity (usually more than four per ten high-power fields), necrosis and large size (>10 cm). Increased mitotic activity and necrosis are the most useful of these criteria. Malignant localized fibrous tumours may have areas that look completely benign, so large tumours should be sampled liberally, (at least one section per centimeter of the tumour diameter) especially from grossly necrotic or haemorrhagic areas.

2.2   Epithelioid hemangioendothelioma
(Figs. 81, 82)

A vascular tumour composed of short cords and nests of epithelioid endothelial cells embedded in a myxohyaline matrix. The tumours are distinctive for their epithelioid character, sharply defined cytoplasmic vacuoles, intraalveolar and intravascular growth and central hyaline necrosis.

Epithelioid hemangioendothelioma [previously called intravascular sclerosing bronchioloalveolar tumour (IVBAT) in the lung] is a low grade angiosarcoma that typically presents in the lung as multiple nodules having a chondroid gross appearance. Up to one third of cases present as a solitary nodule. Rare cases have a pseudomesotheliomatous growth pattern. Epithelioid hemangioendothelioma occurs in a variety of other sites such as the liver, soft tissue and bone. It may present in multiple organs simultaneously.

2.3   Pleuropulmonary blastoma (Figs. 83–85)

A cystic and/or solid sarcoma in which the cystic component is lined by benign metaplastic epithelium that may be ciliated.

When these neoplasms are exclusively cystic, the malignant component consists of primitive small cells beneath the epithelium with the cambium layer-like appearance seen in sarcoma botryoides. Focal rhabdomyoblasts may be found among the malignant small cells. Solid areas have differentiated and/or anaplastic sarcomatous elements including embryonal rhabdomyosarcoma, fibrosarcoma, chondrosarcoma, anaplastic undifferentiated sarcoma and mixtures thereof. Solid islands of primitive cells separated by a myxoid spindle cell stroma may resemble the blastema in Wilms tumour.

Pleuropulmonary blastoma is a dysontogenic malignant neoplasm of early childhood that may involve the lung and/or pleura. Cystic pleuropulmonary blastoma may mimic benign cystic lung disease and hamartomatous lesions. A family history of similar-appearing intrathoracic tumours, other solid tumours of childhood and various malformations is present in up to 30% of cases. This tumour must be distinguished from *pulmonary blastoma* (see Sect. 1.3.6.3) which characteristically occurs in adults. Favourable prognosis correlates with the extent of cystic change.

2.4   Chondroma (Fig. 86)

A benign tumour composed of hyaline or myxohyaline cartilage.

Chondromas of the lung lack the epithelial-lined clefts and admixtures of mesenchymal elements seen in chondroid hamartomas. Metaplastic bone is often seen. Most occur in the setting of the Carney triad [pulmonary chondroma(s), epithelioid smooth muscle tumour(s) of the stomach and extraadrenal paraganglioma(s)] as a single, or occasionally multiple, nodules.

2.5 Calcifying fibrous pseudotumour of the pleura (Fig. 87)

A slow-growing plaque-like lesion occurring in the visceral pleura, composed of nearly acellular fibrous tissue and associated with extensive dystrophic calcification (which may be psammomatous).

2.6 Congenital peribronchial myofibroblastic tumour (Figs. 88, 89)

An interstitial and peribronchovascular proliferation of uniform myofibroblastic cells; cellularity and mitotic activity may be marked.

The prognosis for this lesion (which has also been called congenital leiomyosarcoma and/or fibrosarcoma) appears to be favourable when the tumour is solitary. However, multifocal tumours in the lung of a neonate should suggest the presence of congenital generalized myofibromatosis, which has a poor clinical outcome.

2.7 Diffuse pulmonary lymphangiomatosis (Figs. 90, 91)

A diffuse proliferation of well-formed lymphatic vascular channels, with or without a minor smooth muscle component, affecting lymphatic routes of the lung (pleural, septal, bronchovascular).

In contrast to lymphangioleiomyomatosis, the smooth muscle component (when present) is HMB-45-negative, both sexes are affected and the patients do not have emphysema-like cysts of the lung on chest radiographs.

Affected patients are generally children with interstitial lung disease; associated pleural effusions and mediastinal involvement are common.

2.8 Desmoplastic round cell tumour (Figs. 92, 93)

A malignant tumour composed of irregular cell nests in a dense fibrous or cellular spindle cell stroma. The cells are small to intermediate in size with scant cytoplasm and some nuclear molding. This neoplasm typically shows immunohistochemical evidence of both epithelial (cytokeratin-positive) and muscle (desmin-positive) differentiation.

It is usually encountered as a peritoneal tumour in adolescents and young adults. Pleural and pulmonary involvement is rare.

2.9   Others

3   Mesothelial Tumours

These are benign or malignant tumours of the mesothelial lining cells of the pleura.

3.1   Benign

3.1.1   Adenomatoid tumour (Figs. 94, 95)

A small, circumscribed, solitary tumour composed of small cords, tubules or acini of mesothelial cells resembling adenomatoid tumours at other sites.

3.2   Malignant mesothelioma (Figs. 96–106)

A malignant tumour of mesothelial cells showing a variety of histological patterns.

Virtually all mesotheliomas of the pleura have a diffuse growth pattern and involve both the visceral and parietal surfaces as a thick rind. Early pleural involvement in diffuse mesothelioma may manifest as multiple discrete, small nodules or plaques. Rare localized mesotheliomas have been described as solitary pleural-based masses. The histological subtypes are based on the following growth patterns.

3.2.1   Epithelioid mesothelioma (Figs. 96–100)

A pattern consisting of tubules, acini, papillae or sheets of atypical, epithelioid mesothelial cells. (Synonym: Epithelial mesothelioma).

3.2.2   Sarcomatoid mesothelioma (Fig. 101)

A pure spindled pattern resembling a fibrosarcoma or a malignant fibrous histiocytoma. (Synonyms: Sarcomatous, spindle or diffuse malignant fibrous mesothelioma).

3.2.2.1   *Desmoplastic mesothelioma* (Figs. 102, 103)

A sarcomatoid mesothelioma with a predominance (>50%) of dense collagenous stroma and haphazardly arranged slit-like spaces made up of cells with slightly atypical nuclei.

3.2.3   Biphasic mesothelioma (Fig. 104)

A combined epithelioid and sarcomatoid pattern with each comprising at least 10 percent of the tumour.

Larger tumour sampling will increase the ability to detect a biphasic pattern. Separation of reactive fibrous stroma from a sarcomatoid pattern of biphasic messthelioma may be difficult.

3.2.4   Others

There are a number of less common patterns including the presence of heterologous elements [chondroid, osteoblastic (Fig. 105), rhabdomyoblastic, neurogenic sarcoma-like], adenomatoid tumour-like, lymphohistiocytoid (Fig. 106), myxoid stroma deciduoid, multicystic, clear cell, small cell and poorly differentiated or anaplastic variants. Mesotheliomas containing osteoclastic giant cells may be encountered. Histological subtyping of mesotheliomas is influenced by the size of the biopsy sample; more biphasic tumours are diagnosed in larger specimens.

In contrast to reactive mesothelial hyperplasias, malignant epithelial mesotheliomas show increased cellularity, complex growth patterns, cytologic atypia and stromal invasion. Rare mesotheliomas show a predominantly in situ pattern of spread where atypical mesothelial cells line the pleural surface. In such cases a definitive histological diagnosis of malignant mesothelioma rests on the identification of invasive tumour.

Epithelioid malignant mesotheliomas need to be distinguished from adenocarcinomas; histochemistry and immunohistochemistry are useful in this distinction (Table 4, p. 53). Adenocarcinomas may show intracellular mucin (diastase resistant, periodic acid–Schiff-positive) and tend to stain for cytokeratin and at least two of the carcinomatous epitopes, CEA, B72.3, CD-15 (Leu-M1) and BER-EP4. Epithelioid mesotheliomas are rarely mucin-positive, show strong positivity for cytokeratin stains and are usually negative for CEA, B72.3 and Leu-M1. Epithelioid mesotheliomas frequently show a distinctive mem-

Table 4. Immunohistochemistry of pleural lesions[a]

Diagnostic problem	Keratins (LMW/HMW)	CEA	B72.3	Leu-M1	BER-EP4	EMA HMFG-2	Vim	Actin
I. Mesothelial hyperplasia vs	+-++	-	-	-	-	-/+	-/+	-
Epithelioid mesothelioma vs	+-++	-/+	-/+	-/+	-/+	+ (membrane)	+	-/+
Metastatic carcinoma (usually adenocarcinoma)	+-++	+	+	+	+	+ (cytoplasmic)	-/+	-
II. Fibrous pleuritis vs	+	-	-	-	-	-/+	+	+
Sarcomatoid mesothelioma vs	+	-	-	-	-	-/+	+	+/-
Sarcoma (primary or metastatic)	-/+	-	-	-	-	-	+	*

LMW, low molecular weight; HMW, high molecular weight; HMGF, human milk fat globulin; CEA, carcinoembryonic antigen; EMA, epithelial membrane antigen; Vim, vimentin.

-, Negative; +/-, occasionally positive; -/+, usually negative; *, depends on subtype; +, usually positive.

[a]Until recently there has been no immunohistochemical stain that is positive in mesotheliomas and negative in other lesions. HBME-1, Calretinin, and thrombomodulin have shown some promise as being mesothelioma-specific antibodies, but none is, as yet, widely accepted.

brane pattern of staining for epithelial membrane antigen (EMA) and human milk fat globulin-2. Electron microscopy of epithelioid mesotheliomas characteristically shows long bushy microvilli (length more than 10× the width).

Sarcomatoid mesotheliomas must be distinguished from sarcomas and other spindle cell proliferations. The latter are usually localized masses, whereas mesotheliomas tend to involve the pleura in a diffuse fashion. Sarcomatoid mesotheliomas are often positive with keratin stains, whereas soft tissue sarcomas of the chest wall are only rarely keratin-positive. The desmoplastic variant of sarcomatous mesothelioma must be distinguished from chronic fibrosing pleuritis and since both lesions can express low molecular weight cytokeratins, immunohistochemical stains are of restricted value for this discrimination, though they can be very useful to highlight invasion. Features in favour of desmoplastic mesothelioma include storiform pattern, infarct-like necrosis, foci of increased cellularity and atypia, increased number of atypical mitoses and invasion of adjacent structures, particularly the lung or chest wall.

Tumours that simulate mesothelioma include pseudomesotheliomatous adenocarcinoma, epithelioid hemangioendothelioma, thymoma and desmoplastic round cell tumour.

4   Miscellaneous Tumours

4.1   Hamartoma (Figs. 107, 108)

A tumour composed of an abnormal mixture of tissues normally found in the lung.

The majority are peripheral but central bronchi may also be involved. They are usually solitary, but rarely may be multiple. They are well circumscribed and consist of nodules of connective tissue intersected by epithelial clefts. Cartilage is the commonest connective tissue, but there may also be cellular fibrous tissue, which is often myxoid and fat. All these tissues are well-differentiated and show no evidence of malignancy. The epithelial clefts are lined by ciliated columnar epithelium or non-ciliated epithelium and probably represent entrapment of respiratory epithelium.

The traditional term "hamartoma" is retained for this lesion, but several features suggest it is a neoplasm rather than a congenital lesion such as its rarity in childhood, increasing incidence with age and the finding of chromosomal aberrations involving either 12q14–15 or 6p21, indicating a clonal origin.

4.2   Sclerosing hemangioma (Figs. 109–112)

A tumour of uncertain type with a distinctive constellation of histological findings, including solid, papillary, sclerotic and haemorrhagic patterns. Hyperplastic type II pneumocytes line the surface of the papillary structures. The interstitial epithelioid cells are bland and uniform with pale cytoplasm. Cholesterol clefts, chronic inflammation, xanthoma cells, hemosiderin, calcification, laminated scroll-like whorls, necrosis and mature fat may be seen.

Despite ongoing debate about its histogenesis, the most recent immunohistochemical and ultrastructural data suggest that it is an epithelial tumour. The interstitial polygonal epithelioid cells, possibly of pneumocyte origin, are thought to be the neoplastic cells. These epithelioid tumour cells are often negative for keratin but positive for epithelial membrane antigen. Rarely, neuroendocrine cell hyperplasia or tumourlets are seen within sclerosing hemangiomas. The tumours may be multiple. A neoplastic nature is supported by the rare metastases to hilar lymph nodes and recent molecular studies indicating a clonal origin. More than 80% of patients with sclerosing hemangioma are women. Sclerosing hemangioma is not an unusual tumour in Japan where it is seen as frequently as carcinoid tumours. (*Synonyms*: sclerosing pneumocytoma, sclerosing angioma.)

4.3   Clear cell tumour (Figs. 113–116)

A tumour composed of cells with clear or eosinophilic cytoplasm, which contains abundant glycogen. Thin-walled blood vessels without a muscular coat are characteristic.

Virtually all clear cell tumours are benign and cured by surgical excision. The histogenesis is uncertain. By immunohistochemistry, most clear cell tumours show strong staining for HMB-45 (Fig. 116) and negative staining for keratin. A characteristic ultrastructural feature of clear cell tumour is the presence of abundant cytoplasmic glycogen (Figs. 114 and 115), including intralysosomal glycogen; a small percentage of cells contain recognizable melanosomes. Clear cell tumours have also been reported in the trachea, pancreas and liver. A very rare association with tuberous sclerosis and other HMB-45-positive lesions including angiomyolipoma and lymphangioleiomy-omatosis has been noted. (*Synonym*: sugar tumour.)

4.4   Germ cell tumours

4.4.1   Teratoma, mature (Figs. 117, 118)

4.4.2   Teratoma, immature

A tumour containing tissues representing all three germ cell layers or a dermoid cyst consisting entirely of ectodermal tissue.

To establish that a teratoma is primary in the lung, the tumour should be entirely intrapulmonary without involvement of the mediastinum and there should not be evidence of a gonadal or extragonadal primary. Histologically, most pulmonary teratomas are composed of mature, often cystic somatic tissue, although malignant or immature elements may occur. Mature teratomas of the lung generally take the form of squamous-lined cysts similar to those of the ovary, also known as dermoid cysts. Pancreatic and thymic tissue commonly occur. Metastatic germ cell neoplasms to the lung may consist of only mature teratomatous tissues after chemotherapy and rarely they present as a solitary lung mass.

4.4.3   Other germ cell tumours

Germ cell malignancies other than immature teratomas are extremely rare and require exclusion of an extrapulmonary primary. They should also be distinguished from carcinomas of the lung (including pleomorphic and giant cell carcinomas), which are producing alpha-fetoprotein, chorionic gonadotrophins or placental lactogen.

Most cases reported as choriocarcinoma of the lung are pleomorphic carcinomas with ectopic beta-HCG production. Instead of a dual population of cytotrophoblasts and syncytiotrophoblasts typical of choriocarcinoma, there is a continuous spectrum of morphology from large to pleomorphic tumour cells.

4.5   Thymoma (Figs. 119, 120)

A tumour of the lung or pleura that is histologically identical to mediastinal thymoma.

Radiographic studies and/or surgical inspection must exclude a primary mediastinal tumour. Myasthenia gravis can occur in association with pulmonary thymomas.

4.6   **Malignant melanoma** (Figs. 121, 122)

Nearly all malignant melanomas in the lung are metastatic. Primary melanomas of the lung are extremely rare and show histological and immunohistological features of malignant melanomas as seen elsewhere. To designate a malignant melanoma as primary in the lung, there should be evidence of activity in the bronchial mucosa, transmigration in bronchial epithelium by melanoma cells, an associated solitary mass with morphologic features of a melanoma, no history of prior melanoma and no demonstrable melanoma elsewhere in the body (ideally by a thorough autopsy examination).

Potential occult sites such as the eye and genital tract should be examined.

Tumours that fulfill these criteria may be pigmented or non-pigmented, sessile or polypoid growths involving the large airways. Junctional activity in the bronchial mucosa may also be seen in metastatic melanoma.

4.7   **Others**

Other tumours described as arising in the lung include ependymoma and paraganglioma.

A paraganglioma-like morphology may be seen in carcinoid tumours and most reported paragangliomas of lung are probably carcinoid tumours. Keratin positivity favours a carcinoid since paragangliomas are negative, but not all carcinoids stain for keratin. S-100-positive sustentacular cells may also be seen in carcinoids. What was called paraganglioma (chemodectoma) in the 1981 classification is now known to represent the "multiple meningothelioid nodules" discussed in Sect. 8.2[3]. The following criteria can be used for a diagnosis of pulmonary paraganglioma: (1) A diffuse zellenballen pattern throughout; (2) absence of distinctive features of carcinoids (trabecu-

---

[3]World Health Organization (1981) Histological typing of lung tumors, 2nd edn. WHO, Geneva

lar pattern, pseudoglandular acini, ossification, perivascular pseudorosettes, oncocytic change, spindle cells); (3) presence of distinctive features of paragangliomas (cytoplasmic vacuoles, cell-in-cell embracing phenomenon); (4) absence of immunohistochemical staining for keratin; and (5) absence of a primary paraganglioma elsewhere.

5   Lymphoproliferative Diseases

A number of proliferative lesions of lymphoid cells can present in and remain restricted to the lung for months or years. They may be solitary, multifocal or diffuse. The lung is also frequently involved in disseminated hematolymphoid lesions, both at presentation and at relapse. Some of the pulmonary lymphoid lesions deserve separate comment.

5.1   Lymphoid interstitial pneumonia (LIP)

A diffuse interstitial lymphoid infiltrate.

Two overlapping patterns are recognized: diffuse hyperplasia of lymphoid tissue along bronchovascular bundles, in the pleura and in the septa (diffuse lymphoid hyperplasia); and dense diffuse interstitial infiltrates of lymphocytes and plasma cells which are histologically heterogeneous and immunologically polyclonal. Granulomas may be present.

LIP presents with clinical, radiographic, and often functional features of interstitial lung disease. LIP has been relatively frequently recognized in the setting of HIV infection, other immunodeficiency states and autoimmune diseases. Many cases previously classified as LIP are now recognized as diffuse lymphomas (see Section 5.3). [*Synonyms*: diffuse hyperplasia of bronchial-associated lymphoid tissue (BALT), follicular bronchiolitis.]

5.2   Nodular lymphoid hyperplasia

A localized lesion with abundant lymphoid tissue, usually with associated fibrosis, showing features of reactive lymphoid hyperplasia such as germinal centre formation.

The lymphoid infiltrates consist of polyclonal plasma cells and histiocytes (which may occasionally form granulomas). Light chain restriction and aberrant T-cell phenotypes are not found. (*Synonyms*: pseudolymphoma, nodular lymphoid hyperplasia of BALT.)

Most cases of nodular lymphoid hyperplasia (pseudolymphoma) have been reclassified as low-grade lymphomas of mucosa-associated lymphoid tissue (MALT), and the existence of this category has been questioned.

5.3   Low-grade marginal zone B-cell lymphoma of the mucosa-associated lymphoid tissue (MALT) (Figs. 123, 124)

A malignant lymphoma that reflects features of normal MALT or BALT, including the presence of residual germinal centres, plasma cells (which may be polyclonal or monoclonal), and atypical small lymphocytes which may resemble monocytoid B cells or cleaved cells.

Infiltration of bronchial or bronchiolar epithelium (lymphoepithelial lesions) is characteristic. Some cases may be associated with varying degrees of fibrosis and granuloma formation.

Phenotyping shows light chain restriction in the small B-lymphocytes and sometimes in the plasma cell component. Some cases have large numbers of T-lymphocytes.

Most cases previously interpreted as pseudolymphomas of the lung are now recognized as low-grade lymphomas of MALT. These lesions may form solitary nodules or infiltrates, multiple nodules or infiltrates or diffuse bilateral infiltrates. Histologically the appearance of these low-grade lymphomas is produced by a mixture of small lymphocytes, often with plasma cells, centrocyte-like cells and monocytoid B-cells, and ill-formed granulomas. The tumours tend to invade along lymphatic pathways, penetrating the pleura in a plaque-like fashion, and bronchial cartilage.

5.4   Lymphomatoid granulomatosis (Figs. 125-127)

A malignant lymphoma featuring a polymorphous angiocentric lymphoid infiltrate with central necrosis and prominent infiltration of vessels by lymphoid cells.

The lesions are histologically heterogeneous and contain variable numbers of atypical large cells (some histologically qualify as diffuse large cell lymphoma) which usually stain as B-cells and small lymphocytes that stain as T-cells. Plasma cells are inconspicuous. Epithelioid histiocytes may be prominent. Sarcoid-like granulomas and giant cells are unusual. (*Synonyms*: angiocentric lymphoma, angioimmuno-proliferative lesion.)

Lymphomatoid granulomatosis has been recognized as a lympho-proliferative disease. These are now regarded as diffuse large B-cell lymphomas which vary in the number of admixed T-cells and in the histologic grade. The neoplastic cell is a large B-cell that may be shown to be clonal and to contain Epstein-Barr virus. Some cases that show histologic features resembling lymphomatoid granulomatosis have been shown to be T-cell lymphomas. Lymphomatoid granulo-matosis can present as a solitary mass or as multiple bilateral nodules with central necrosis and cavitation.

6   Secondary Tumours

The lung is the most common site of metastasis in the body and metas-tases may mimic primary tumours of the lung. Metastases to the lung may show the following patterns: solitary nodule, multiple nodules (with or wthout cavitation), endobronchial, pleural, intra-arterial tumour emboli (with or without infarction, with or without cor pul-monale), lymphangitic (within lymphatic vessels or growing along lymphatic routes in the pleura, septa, and around bronchovascular structures), lepidic (lining alveolar walls), pneumonic consolidation and mixtures of the above.

Foci of lepidic growth similar to bronchioloalveolar carcinoma are seen occasionally with metastatic carcinomas and may be associated with any of the patterns listed above. Cavitation and cystic change (especially in metastatic low grade sarcomas) may be associated with pneumothorax and mimic cystic lung diseases. Interstitial growth by metastatic neoplasms may be marked, particularly in the case of some metastatic sarcomas.

A number of tumours generally considered benign may occasion-ally develop lung metastases: uterine smooth muscle tumours (so-called benign metastasizing leiomyoma), thymomas, pleomorphic ade-nomas of salivary-gland origin, meningioma, chondroblastoma and giant cell tumour of bone.

Benign metastasizing leiomyoma (Figs. 128, 129) is a distinctive clinicopathologic condition seen almost exclusively in women who typically present with multiple slow-growing lung nodules composed of benign-appearing smooth muscle. Most have concomitant uterine leiomyomas or give a history of hysterectomy for leiomyomas. The nodules are generally solid and composed of benign-appearing smooth muscle cells that may be associated with secondary cystic change in which the cysts are lined by metaplastic epithelium. Most reported examples of multifocal leiomyomatous hamartomas of the lung represent benign metastasizing leiomyoma. Cellular examples of benign metastasizing leiomyoma are histologically (and conceptually) difficult to separate from metastatic low-grade leiomyosarcoma.

7   Unclassified Tumours

Tumours that cannot be placed in any of the above listed categories.

8   Tumour-Like Lesions

8.1   Tumourlet (Figs. 130, 131)

A microscopic, peribronchiolar, nodular aggregate of uniform, round to oval or spindle-shaped cells with moderate amounts of cytoplasm and morphology similar to the cells of carcinoid tumours.

These lesions may be multiple and are usually a chance microscopic finding in scarred lungs, particularly those affected by bronchiectasis. Immunohistochemistry and electron microscopy have shown that the cells are neuroendocrine. The unwary pathologist may mistake them for small cell carcinoma, from which they differ in the regularity of their nuclei and lack of mitotic activity. If such neuroendocrine cell aggregates are palpable or can be discerned by the naked eye they are more likely to be carcinoid tumours (see Sect. 1.3.7). Lesions 0.5 cm or greater are arbitrarily called carcinoid tumours. Neuroendocrine cell hyperplasia may be seen in the adjacent bronchiolar mucosa. Tumourlets are generally an incidental pathological curiosity of no clinical importance, but in a few cases with diffuse neuroendocrine cell hyperplasia they have been associated with obliterative bronchiolar fibrosis and obstructive airways disease. It has been suggested that the neuroendocrine cells may cause bronchiolar scarring by secreting fibrogenic substances.

8.2   Minute meningothelioid nodule
(Figs. 132, 133)

Perivenular nodular aggregates of small regular cells that are entirely interstitial and have no contact with the air spaces (previously known as multiple minute chemodectomas).

The cells are often in "zellballen"-like arrangements that are reminiscent of chemodectomas. They have a moderate amount of cytoplasm and their nuclei are round to oval with finely granular chromatin. Intranuclear cytoplasmic inclusions are frequent. Electron microscopy and immunohistochemistry have shown that the cells resemble meningothelial cells rather than chemoreceptor cells. The lesions are usually multiple and chance microscopic findings of no clinical importance.

These tumours were classified as paragangliomas in the 1981 classification (see Sect. 4.7)[4].

8.3   Langerhans cell histiocytosis
(Langerhans cell granulomatosis, eosinophilic granuloma, histiocytosis X) (Figs. 134, 135)

A diffuse, bilateral, multinodular interstitial infiltrate of Langerhans cells with an ill-defined cell border, a reniform, vesicular nucleus and a moderate amount of eosinophilic cytoplasm that lacks evidence of phagocytic activity. The Langerhans cells are generally mixed with plentiful eosinophils.

The infiltrate is generally centered on bronchioles and destruction of these leads to focal scars or cystic change. Eventually, lymphocytes and pigment-laden macrophages replace the Langerhans cells and eosinophils. At this stage the lesions lack specific features, but the scars have a characteristic stellate outline.

Langerhans cells stain immunohistochemically with antibodies for S-100 protein and/or CD1a.

Pulmonary disease may be the only manifestation of Langerhans cell histiocytosis or the lungs may be involved as part of a generalized disease. Patients with pulmonary involvement generally develop restrictive lung disease and may develop pneumothoraces. Adult

---

[4]World Health Organization (1981) Histological typing of lung tumors, 2nd edn. WHO, Geneva

patients with pulmonary involvement are usually cigarette smokers. The condition is more likely to be mistaken for a fibroinflammatory or lymphoproliferative condition than a tumour.

8.4 Inflammatory pseudotumour (inflammatory myofibroblastic tumour)
(Figs. 136–139)

A spectrum of fibroblastic or myofibroblastic proliferations with a varying infiltrate of inflammatory cells, typically plasma cells, lymphocytes, and/or foamy histiocytes. The lesions may range from a primarily myofibroblastic or fibroxanthomatous appearance to one that has a heavy infiltrate of plasma cells.

These lesions are usually solitary but multicentric examples have been described. This is one of the most common lung tumours in children, but it can occur at any age. They are well circumscribed but lack a capsule. Recurrence following surgery is uncommon. If the lesion has reached the mediastinum or chest wall complete excision may not be possible. In such cases the usual excellent prognosis is transformed by slow progressive infiltration of these tissues. The reactive vs neoplastic nature of this condition has not been entirely settled. As the tumours may show mitoses, necrosis, vascular invasion and infiltration of the chest wall or mediastinal structures, they should be differentiated if possible from fibrous histiocytoma and sarcomatoid carcinoma, especially in adults. This distinction may be difficult. (*Synonyms*: inflammatory myofibroblastic tumor, plasma cell granuloma, fibroxanthoma, fibrous histiocytoma, pseudosarcomatous myofibroblastic tumour, and invasive fibrous tumour of the tracheobronchial tree.)

8.5 Localized organizing pneumonia (Fig. 140)

A discrete nodule in which alveoli and respiratory bronchioles are filled by polypoid knots of myxoid granulation tissue (Masson bodies).

This histological pattern is non-specific and can be seen in a wide variety of settings, including a solitary coin lesion which is often excised under the suspicion of malignancy. While the lesion may appear discrete on gross and radiologic examination, this feature may be less striking on histological examination. More often, organizing pneumonia is multifocal and raises the differential diagnosis of cryptogenic organizing pneumonia (also known as idiopathic bronchiolitis obliterans organizing pneumonia). If neutrophils are present, this probably represents an organizing acute pneumonia or an organizing abscess, but the distinction between these two entities is not always straightforward.

8.6   Amyloid tumour (nodular amyloid) (Fig. 141)

A tumour-like lesion consisting of eosinophilic amorphous deposits of amyloid, generally attended by a lymphoplasmacytic infiltrate and foreign body giant cells.

Amyloid tumours may be solitary or multiple and may be found in any part of the lower respiratory tract from the trachea to the pleura. Apple-green birefringence is characteristic with the Congo-red stain. They differ from pulmonary involvement by systemic amyloid, which takes the form of diffuse thickening of the alveolar walls. Amyloid may be seen in lymphomas and carcinoids. Rarely, light-microscopically similar masses can be produced by deposits of light chains (so-called light chain disease), but these deposits lack Congophilia.

8.7   Hyalinizing granuloma (Fig. 142)

A nodule of hyaline collagen that may be solitary or multiple.

The collagen bundles often form broad bands. Chronic inflammation may be prominent at the periphery but it is usually mild or moderate within the lesion. It may be associated with granulomatous inflammation, sclerosing mediastinitis, retroperitoneal fibrosis or Riedel thyroiditis.

8.8   Lymphangioleiomyomatosis (Figs. 143, 144)

A widespread interstitial infiltrate of immature short spindle cells resembling smooth muscle cells and associated with cystic change.

Cystic change is usually a striking feature. The distinctive immature smooth muscle cells often form microscopic nodules in the walls of the cysts. These cells have properties of smooth muscle cells by electron microscopy and immunohistochemistry and stain for HMB-45. The infiltrate may also involve pulmonary venules, obstructing them to cause capillary haemorrhage, with resultant hemosiderosis.

This condition occurs in women primarily in the reproductive years. It may occur in isolation or be part of a wider process that also includes lymph nodes and lymphatics of the trunk. It may also be a manifestation of tuberous sclerosis in women. The condition is progressive and generally results in death from respiratory failure several years after onset unless the menopause is first reached or oestrogen antagonists arrest progression.

8.9   Micronodular pneumocyte hyperplasia
(Figs. 145, 146)

A multifocal micronodular proliferation of type II cells with mild thickening of the interstitium.

This condition is extremely rare and is most frequently seen in patients with tuberous sclerosis and also often associated with lymphangioleiomyomatosis. The lesions are generally less than 5 mm in size.

8.10   Endometriosis (Figs. 147, 148)

This may rarely present as a nodular intrapulmonary mass (an endometrioma) or, more commonly, affect the pleura. The former may cause catamenial hemoptysis and the latter may cause catamenial pneumothorax.

Pleuropulmonary endometriosis is encountered most often in women of childbearing age, but it can occur in older women on hormone replacement therapy. Haemorrhage is often present histologically. Rarely, during pregnancy the stroma may undergo extensive decidualization.

8.11   Bronchial inflammatory polyp (Figs. 149, 150)

A fibroinflammatory polyp consisting of oedematous stroma lined by respiratory epithelium that may show squamous metaplasia. Acute and/or chronic inflammation is a prominent feature. Granulation tissue may be seen.

8.12　Others

A variety of other lesions may resemble tumours clinically. Foremost among these are infective conditions such as tuberculosis and the mycoses. Among other less common tumour-like lesions are the non-infective granulomatoses (Wegener granulomatosis, nodular sarcoid, Churg-Strauss angiitis and granulomatosis, bronchocentric granulomatosis, rheumatoid nodules), parasitic infestation, bronchogenic cyst, congenital cystic adenomatoid malformation, sequestration and rounded atelectasis.

TNM Classification of Lung Carcinoma[1]

Rules for Classification

The classification applies only to carcinomas. There should be histological confirmation of the disease and division of cases by histological type.

The following are the procedures for assessing T, N and M categories:

T categories	Physical examination, imaging, endoscopy, and/or surgical exploration
N categories	Physical examination, imaging, endoscopy, and/or surgical exploration
M categories	Physical examination, imaging, and/or surgical exploration

Anatomical Subsites

1. Main bronchus (C34.0)
2. Upper lobe (C34.1)
3. Middle lobe (C34.2)
4. Lower lobe (C34.3)

Regional Lymph Nodes

The regional lymph nodes are the intrathoracic, scalene and supraclavicular nodes.

[1]Sobin LH, Wittekind Ch (eds) (1997) TNM classification of malignant tumours, 5th edn. Wiley, New York, pp 93–100

TNM Clinical Classification

T – Primary Tumour

TNM Categories

TX   Primary tumour cannot be assessed, or tumour proven by the presence of malignant cells in sputum or bronchial washings, but not visualized by imaging or bronchoscopy

T0   No evidence of primary tumour

Tis   Carcinoma in situ

T1   Tumour 3 cm or less in greatest dimension, surrounded by lung or visceral pleura, without bronchoscopic evidence of invasion more proximal than the lobar bronchus (i.e., not in the main bronchus)[a]

T2   Tumour with any of the following features of size or extent:
More than 3 cm in greatest dimension
Involves main bronchus, 2 cm or more distal to the carina
Invades visceral pleura
Associated with atelectasis or obstructive pneumonitis that extends to the hilar region, but does not involve the entire lung

T3   Tumour of any size that directly invades any of the following: chest wall (including superior sulcus tumours), diaphragm, mediastinal pleura, parietal pericardium; or tumour in the main bronchus less than 2 cm distal to the carina[a]–, but without involvement of the carina; or associated atelectasis or obstructive pneumonitis of the entire lung

T4   Tumour of any size that invades any of the following: mediastinum, heart, great vessels, trachea, oesophagus, vertebral body, carina; separate tumour nodule(s) in the same lobe; tumour with malignant pleural effusion[b]

---

[a] The uncommon superficial spreading tumour of any size with its invasive component limited to the bronchial wall, which may extend proximal to the main bronchus, is also classified as T1.

[b] Most pleural effusions with lung cancer are due to tumour. In a few patients, however, multiple cytopathological examinations of pleural fluid are negative for tumour, and the fluid is non-bloody and is not an exudate. Where these elements and clinical judgment dictate that the effusion is not related to the tumour, the effusion should be excluded as a staging element and the patient should be classified as T1, T2 or T3.

N – Regional Lymph Nodes

NX   Regional lymph nodes cannot be assessed
N0   No regional lymph node metastasis
N1   Metastasis in ipsilateral peribronchial
          and/or ipsilateral hilar lymph nodes and intrapulmonary
          nodes, including involvement by direct extension
N2   Metastasis in ipsilateral mediastinal and/or subcarinal
          lymph node(s)
N3   Metastasis in contralateral mediastinal, contralateral
          hilar, ipsilateral or contralateral scalene or
          supraclavicular lymphnode(s)

M – Distant Metastasis

MX   Distant metastasis cannot be assessed
M0   No distant metastasis
M1   Distant metastasis, includes separate tumour nodule(s) in
          a different lobe (ipsilateral or contralateral)

pTNM Pathological Classification

The pT, pN and pM categories correspond to the T, N and M categories.
pN0   Histological examination of hilar and mediastinal lymphadenectomy specimen(s) will ordinarily include six or more lymph nodes.

G – Histopathological Grading

GX   Grade of differentiation cannot be assessed
GI   Well differentiated
G2   Moderately differentiated
G3   Poorly differentiated
G4   Undifferentiated

Stage Grouping

Occult carcinoma	TX	N0	M0
Stage 0	Tis	N0	M0
Stage IA	T1	N0	M0
Stage IB	T2	N0	M0
Stage IIA	T1	N1	M0
Stage IIB	T2	N1	M0
	T3	N0	M0
Stage IIIA	T1	N2	M0
	T2	N2	M0
	T3	N1, N2	M0
Stage IIIB	Any T	N3	M0
	T4	Any N	M0
Stage IV	Any T	Any N	M1

TNM Classification of Malignant Mesothelioma of the Pleura

Rules for Classification

The classification applies only to malignant mesothelioma of the pleura. There should be histological confirmation of the disease.

The following are the procedures for assessing T, N and M categories:

T categories	Physical examination, imaging, endoscopy and/or surgical exploration
N categories	Physical examination, imaging, endoscopy and/or surgical exploration
M categories	Physical examination, imaging and/or surgical exploration

Regional Lymph Nodes

The regional lymph nodes are the intrathoracic, scalene and supraclavicular nodes.

TNM Clinical Classification

T – Primary Tumour

TX	Primary tumour cannot be assessed
T0	No evidence of primary tumour
T1	Tumour limited to ipsilateral parietal and/or visceral pleura
T2	Tumour invades any of the following: ipsilateral lung, endothoracic fascia, diaphragm, pericardium
T3	Tumour invades any of the following: ipsilateral chest wall muscle, ribs, mediastinal organs or tissues

T4   Tumour directly extends to any of the following:
            contralateral pleura, contralateral lung, peritoneum,
            intraabdominal organs, cervical tissues

N – Regional Lymph Nodes

NX   Regional lymph nodes cannot be assessed
N0   No regional lymph node metastasis
N1   Metastasis in ipsilateral peribronchial and/or ipsilateral
            hilar lymph nodes, including involvement by direct
            extension
N2   Metastasis in ipsilateral mediastinal and/or subcarinal
            lymph node(s)
N3   Metastasis in contralateral mediastinal, contralateral
            hilar, ipsilateral or contralateral scalene,
            or supraclavicular lymph node(s)

M – Distant Metastasis

MX   Distant metastasis cannot be assessed
M0   No distant metastasis
Ml   Distant metastasis

pTNM Pathological Classification

The pT, pN and pM categories correspond to the T, N and M categories.

Stage Grouping

Stage I	T1	N0	M0
	T2	N0	M0
Stage II	T1	N1	M0
	T2	N1	M0
Stage III	T1	N2	M0
	T2	N2	M0
	T3	N0, N1, N2	M0
Stage IV	Any T	N3	M0
	T4	Any N	M0
	Any T	Any N	M1

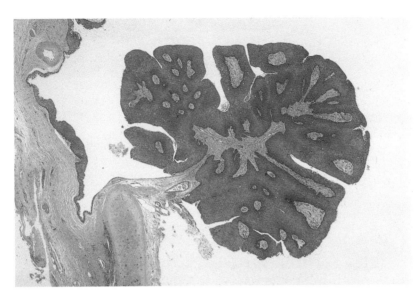

Fig. 1. *Exophytic squamous papilloma.* Mature squamous epithelial cells are growing in an exophytic papillary pattern on the surface of thin fibrovascular cores. The papilloma is attached to the underlying bronchial wall by a stalk
[From Flieder, DB, Koss, MN, Nicholson, A, Sesterhenn, IA, Petras, RE, Travis, WD (1998) Solitary Pulmonary Papillomas in Adults. A Clinicopathologic and in Situ Hybridization Study of 14 Cases Combined With 27 Cases in the Literature, Am. J. Surg. Pathol. 22:1328-1342]

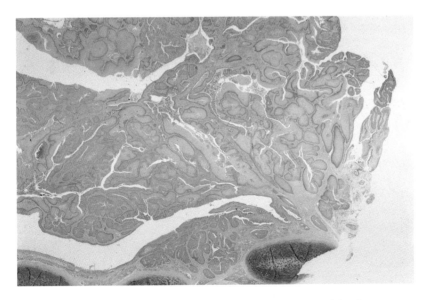

Fig. 2. *Inverted squamous cell papilloma.* Mature squamous epithelial cells are growing in an inverted papillary pattern within the lumen of this bronchus
[From Flieder, DB, Koss, MN, Nicholson, A, Sesterhenn, IA, Petras, RE, Travis, WD (1998) Solitary Pulmonary Papillomas in Adults. A Clinicopathologic and in Situ Hybridization Study of 14 Cases Combined With 27 Cases in the Literature, Am. J. Surg. Pathol. 22:1328-1342]

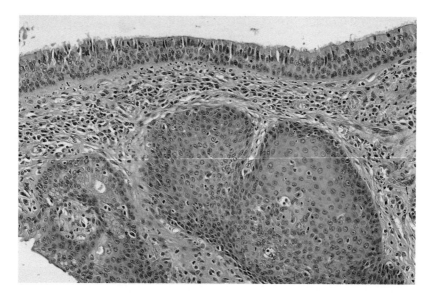

Fig. 3. *Inverted squamous cell papilloma.* Mature squamous cells are growing in a papillary configuration with an inverted pattern of growth
[From Flieder, DB, Koss, MN, Nicholson, A, Sesterhenn, IA, Petras, RE, Travis, WD (1998) Solitary Pulmonary Papillomas in Adults. A Clinicopathologic and in Situ Hybridization Study of 14 Cases Combined With 27 Cases in the Literature, Am. J. Surg. Pathol. 22:1328-1342]

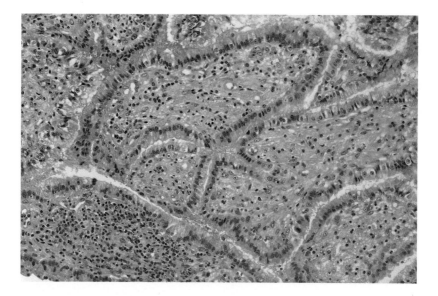

Fig. 4. *Glandular papilloma.* Columnar epithelial cells proliferate in a papillary fashion along the surface of fibrovascular cores
[From Flieder, DB, Koss, MN, Nicholson, A, Sesterhenn, IA, Petras, RE, Travis, WD (1998) Solitary Pulmonary Papillomas in Adults. A Clinicopathologic and in Situ Hybridization Study of 14 Cases Combined With 27 Cases in the Literature, Am. J. Surg. Pathol. 22:1328-1342]

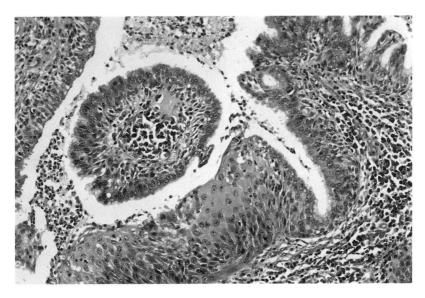

Fig. 5. *Mixed squamous cell and glandular papilloma*
[From Flieder, DB, Koss, MN, Nicholson, A, Sesterhenn, IA, Petras, RE, Travis, WD
(1998) Solitary Pulmonary Papillomas in Adults. A Clinicopathologic and in Situ
Hybridization Study of 14 Cases Combined With 27 Cases in the Literature, Am. J.
Surg. Pathol. 22:1328-1342]

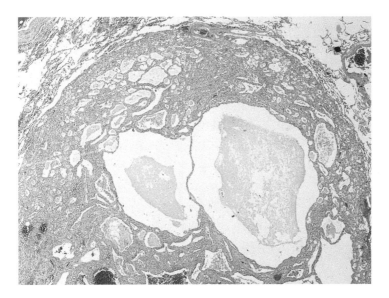

Fig. 6. *Alveolar adenoma.* This tumour nodule is circumscribed, but not encapsulat-
ed. There are large cysts and smaller spaces resembling alveoli
[From Burke, L, WL, Khoor, A, Mackay, B, Oliveira, P, Whitsett, JA, Singh, G,
Turnicky, R, Fleming, MV, Koss, MN, Travis, WD (1999) Alveolar Adenoma: a
Histochemical, Immunohistochemical and Ultrastructural Analysis of 17 Cases,
Hum. Pathol. 30:158-167]

76

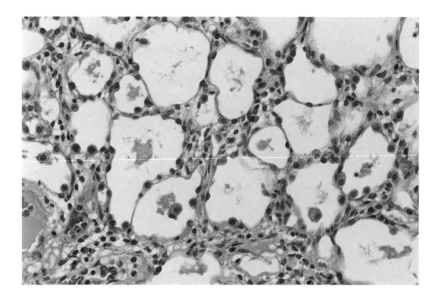

Fig. 7. *Alveolar adenoma.* Alveolus-like spaces are lined by flat or cuboidal pneu-
mocytes on the surface of a thin layer of vascular connective tissue resembling an
alveolar wall. A few macrophages are present within the alveolar-like spaces
[From Burke, L, WL, Khoor, A, Mackay, B, Oliveira, P, Whitsett, JA, Singh, G,
Turnicky, R, Fleming, MV, Koss, MN, Travis, WD (1999) Alveolar Adenoma: a
Histochemical, Immunohistochemical and Ultrastructural Analysis of 17 Cases,
Hum. Pathol. 30:158-167]

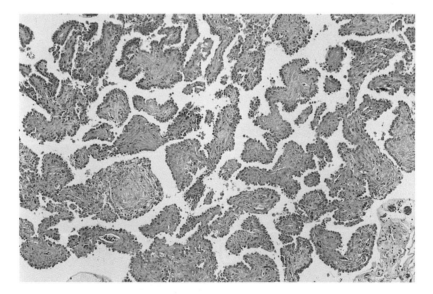

Fig. 8. *Papillary adenoma.* Epithelial cells are growing in a papillary pattern on the
surface of fibrovascular connective tissue

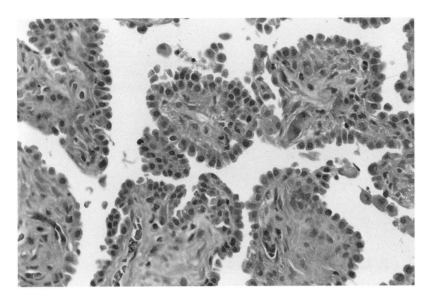

Fig. 9. *Papillary adenoma.* Cuboidal epithelial cells line the surface of the fibrovascular cores

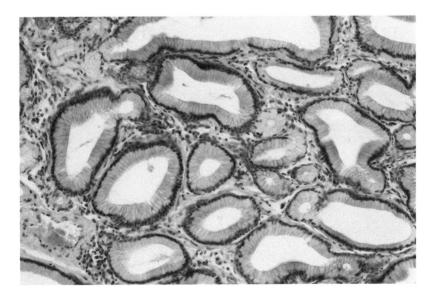

Fig. 10. *Mucous gland adenoma.* The tumour consists entirely of glands lined by columnar epithelium with small basally oriented nuclei and abundant apical mucinous cytoplasm

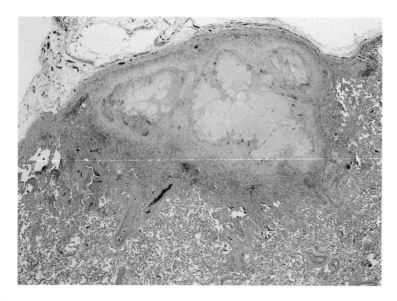

Fig. 11. *Mucinous cystadenoma.* A subpleural cystic tumour is surrounded by a fibrous wall and contains abundant mucus

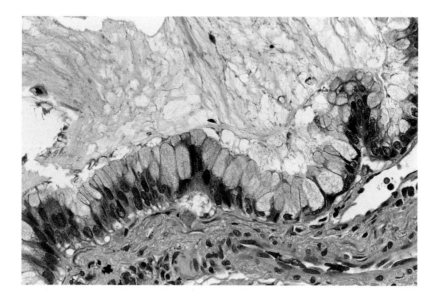

Fig. 12. *Mucinous cystadenoma.* Columnar epithelial cells line the wall of the cyst. Most of the nuclei are basally oriented but there is focal nuclear pseudostratification. The apical cytoplasm is filled with abundant mucin

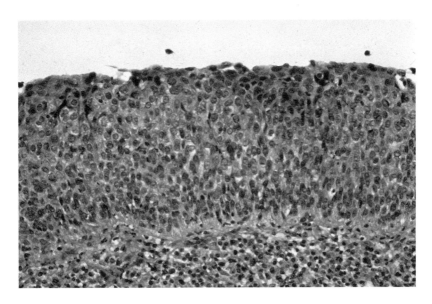

Fig. 13. *Squamous cell carcinoma in situ.* Atypical squamous epithelial cells replacing the full thickness of the mucosa with only focal maturation at the surface

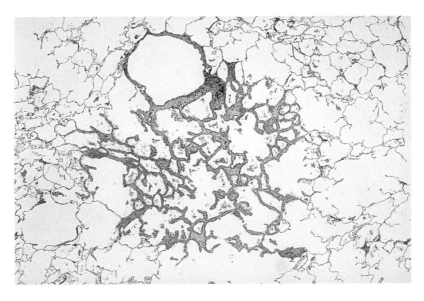

Fig. 14. *Atypical adenomatous hyperplasia.* A small millimeter-sized bronchioloalveolar lesion consists of pneumocytes proliferating in a lepidic fashion along thin alveolar walls. The lesion is situated adjacent to a bronchiole

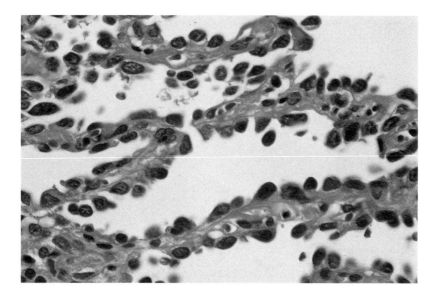

Fig. 15. *Atypical adenomatous hyperplasia.* Cuboidal pneumocytes line the alveolar walls with gaps between the adjacent cells rather than a continuous layer of cells. There is slight thickening of the alveolar walls by fibrous connective tissue, but substantial inflammation or scarring is lacking

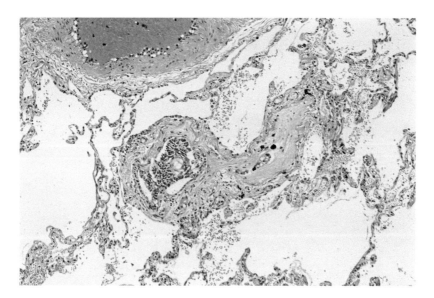

Fig. 16. *Diffuse idiopathic pulmonary neuroendocrine cell hyperplasia.* Fibrous thickening and proliferation of neuroendocrine cells narrow the bronchiole lumen

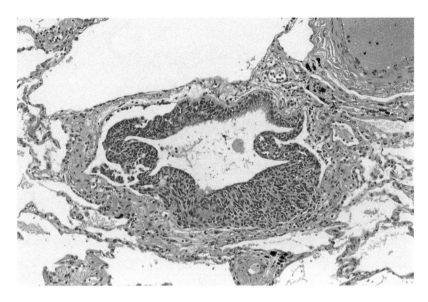

Fig. 17. *Diffuse idiopathic pulmonary neuroendocrine cell hyperplasia.* The bronchiolar epithelium is almost entirely replaced by proliferating neuroendocrine cells

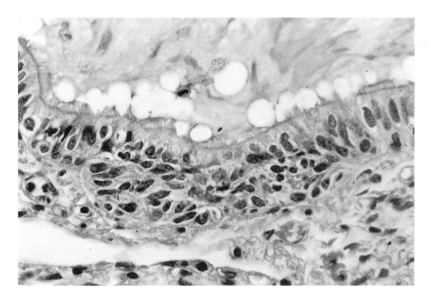

Fig. 18. *Diffuse idiopathic pulmonary neuroendocrine cell hyperplasia.* Hyperplastic neuroendocrine cells form a nest at the base of the bronchiolar epithelium

82

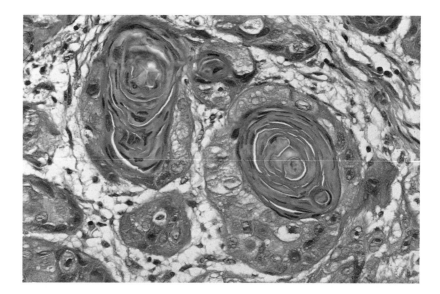

Fig. 19. *Squamous cell carcinoma.* This squamous cell carcinoma is invading a fibrous stroma. Squamous cell differentiation is evident by the keratin pearls and prominent keratinization. Cytologic atypia with hyperchromatic nuclei indicates cytologic malignancy

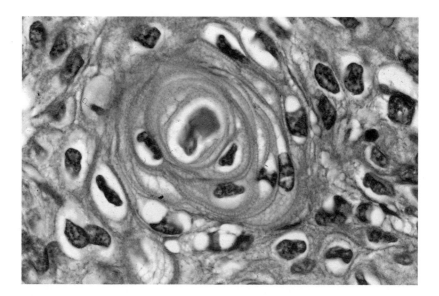

Fig. 20. *Squamous cell carcinoma.* Squamous differentiation, in these cytologically malignant cells, is manifest by the squamous pearl and distinct intercellular bridges

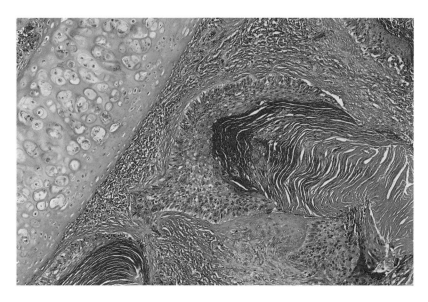

Fig. 21. *Squamous cell carcinoma.* The squamous differentiation of these tumour cells is evident by the many layers of keratin

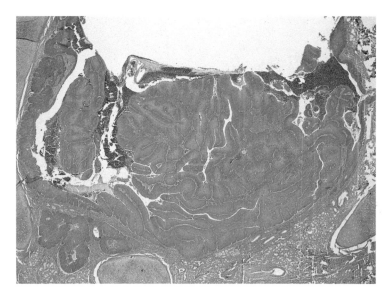

Fig. 22. *Squamous cell carcinoma, papillary variant.* This exophytic, endobronchial squamous cell carcinoma shows a papillary pattern of growth

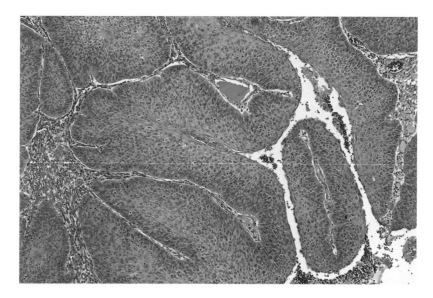

Fig. 23. *Squamous cell carcinoma, papillary variant.* The well-differentiated squamous carcinoma is growing in a papillary pattern

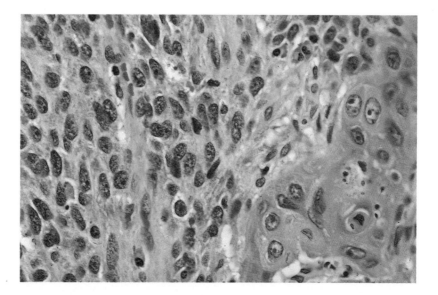

Fig. 24. *Squamous cell carcinoma, small cell variant.* The tumour cells are relatively small with granular nuclear chromatin but there is relatively ample cytoplasm and a few cells with prominent nucleoli

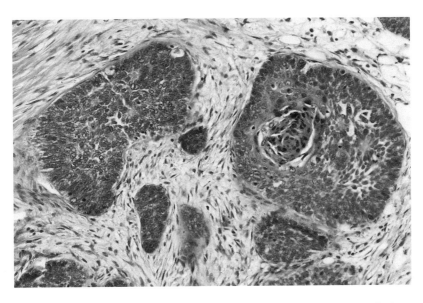

Fig. 25. *Squamous cell carcinoma, basaloid variant.* The nests of tumour cells have prominent peripheral palisading of cells with less cytoplasm and more hyperchromatic nuclei than the tumour cells situated more centrally that have more abundant cytoplasm and prominent keratinization

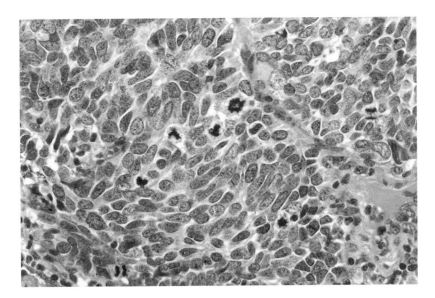

Fig. 26. *Small cell carcinoma.* The tumour cells are densely packed, small, with scant cytoplasm, finely granular nuclear chromatin and absence of nucleoli. Mitoses are frequent

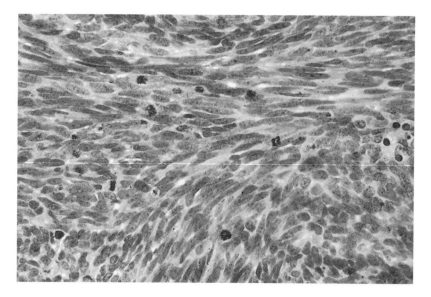

Fig. 27. *Small cell carcinoma.* The fusiform (spindle cell) shape of these cells is a prominent feature in this tumour. Mitoses are frequent and the cells have scant cytoplasm. The nuclear chromatin is finely granular and nucleoli are absent or inconspicuous

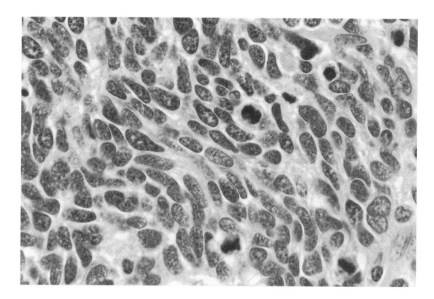

Fig. 28. *Small cell carcinoma.* The cells in this tumour are somewhat larger and show some cytoplasm, as well as a few inconspicuous nucleoli, but otherwise have the cytologic features of small cell carcinoma

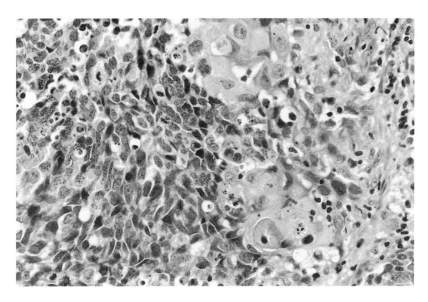

Fig. 29. *Combined small cell and squamous cell carcinoma.* This tumour is composed of a combination of small cell carcinoma and squamous cell carcinoma
[From Colby, TV, Koss, MN, Travis, WD (1995) Tumors of the Lower Respiratory Tract; Atlas of Tumour Pathology, Third Series, Washington, D.C., Armed Forces Institute of Pathology]

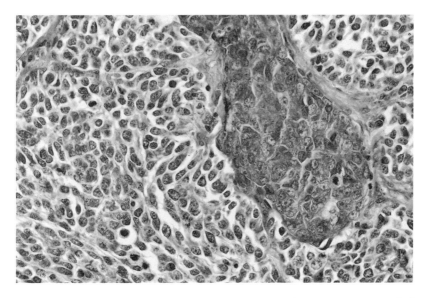

Fig. 30. *Combined small cell and large cell carcinoma.* This tumour is composed of a combination of small cell carcinoma and large cell carcinoma. Most of the tumour consists of small cell carcinoma. The large cell component has cells of larger size with more abundant cytoplasm and prominent nucleoli
[From Colby, TV, Koss, MN, Travis, WD (1995) Tumors of the Lower Respiratory Tract; Atlas of Tumour Pathology, Third Series, Washington, D.C., Armed Forces Institute of Pathology]

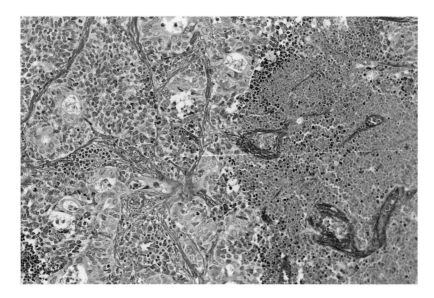

Fig. 31. *Combined small cell and adenocarcinoma.* This tumour consists of small cell carcinoma and adenocarcinoma. Vascular basophilia due to DNA encrustation of the vessel walls is present in the area of tumour necrosis

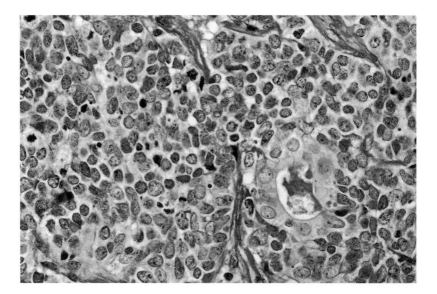

Fig. 32. *Combined small cell and adenocarcinoma.* A malignant gland is present within the small cell carcinoma

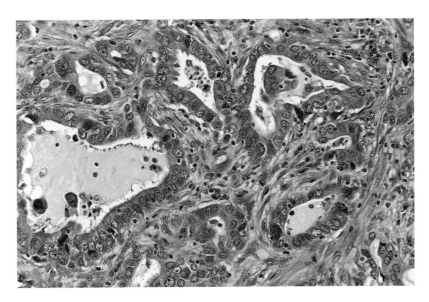

Fig. 33. *Acinar adenocarcinoma.* This tumour forms irregular-shaped glands with cytologically malignant cells exhibiting hyperchromatic nuclei
[From Colby, TV, Koss, MN, Travis, WD (1995) Tumors of the Lower Respiratory Tract; Atlas of Tumour Pathology, Third Series, Washington, D.C., Armed Forces Institute of Pathology]

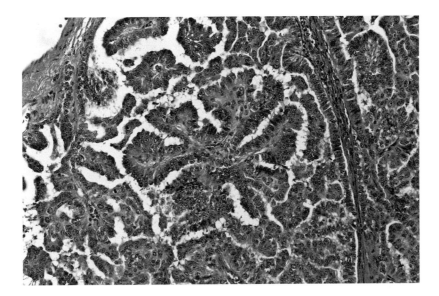

Fig. 34. *Papillary adenocarcinoma.* The tumour cells show a glandular proliferation growing in a papillary pattern along fibrovascular cores

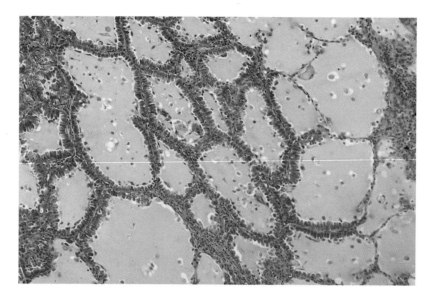

Fig. 35. *Bronchioloalveolar carcinoma, non-mucinous.* These cuboidal- to columnar-shaped cells are growing in a lepidic pattern along the alveolar walls, which maintain the original architecture of the preexisting alveolar parenchyma

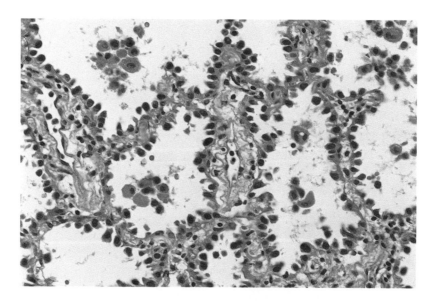

Fig. 36. *Bronchioloalveolar carcinoma, non-mucinous.* The cuboidal- to columnar-shaped cells line the alveolar walls in a lepidic fashion. This morphology is often seen in tumours with type II pneumocyte differentiation

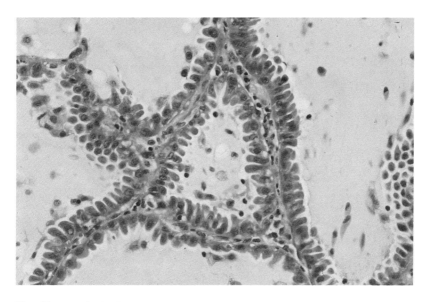

Fig. 37. *Bronchioloalveolar carcinoma, non-mucinous.* The cuboidal- to columnar-shaped cells have basally oriented nuclei and elongated eosinophilic cytoplasm with apical snouts. This is a pattern often seen in tumours with Clara-cell differentiation

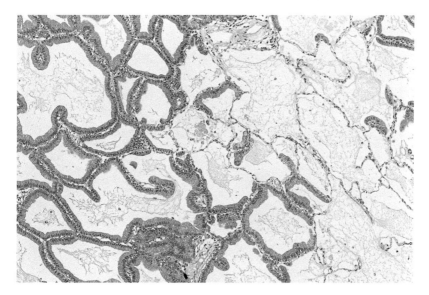

Fig. 38. *Bronchioloalveolar carcinoma, mucinous.* The columnar cells with abundant cytoplasmic mucin are proliferating along the alveolar walls in a lepidic fashion

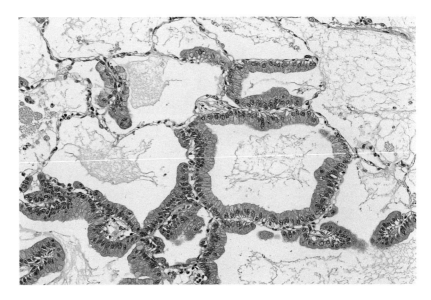

Fig. 39. *Bronchioloalveolar carcinoma, mucinous.* The goblet cells show abundant mucin-rich cytoplasm and the nuclei are small, often situated at the base of the cell

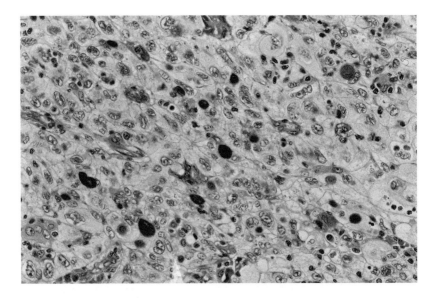

Fig. 40. *Solid adenocarcinoma with mucin.* This poorly differentiated subtype of adenocarcinoma shows a substantial number of intracytoplasmic mucin droplets as seen on this periodic acid-Schiff stain after diastase digestion

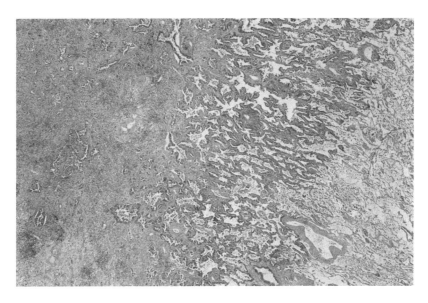

Fig. 41. *Adenocarcinoma, mixed acinar and bronchioloalveolar.* While most of the periphery of the tumour shows a bronchioloalveolar pattern, there is an invasive acinar pattern within the central area of scarring

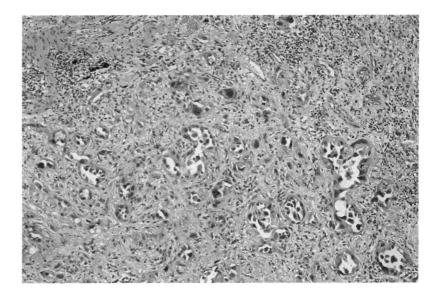

Fig. 42. *Adenocarcinoma, mixed acinar and bronchioloalveolar.* Within the area of scarring this tumour has invasive growth showing infiltrating large atypical malignant cells and a few acini

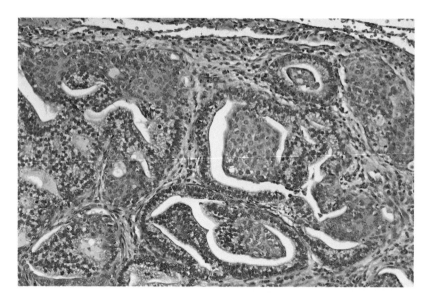

Fig. 43. *Well-differentiated fetal adenocarcinoma.* This tumour grows in glands that have endometrioid morphology. The cells are columnar with clear cytoplasm that often has subnuclear vacuoles similar to endometrial glands. Squamoid morules are present within the glands

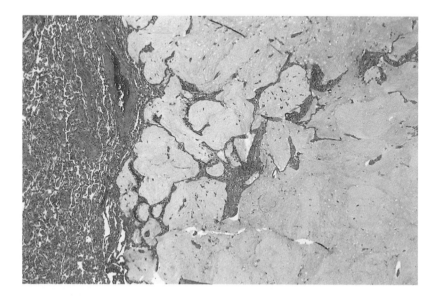

Fig. 44. *Mucinous ("colloid") adenocarcinoma.* This tumour consists of abundant mucin expanding alveolar spaces and spreading in a permeative fashion into adjacent alveolar tissue

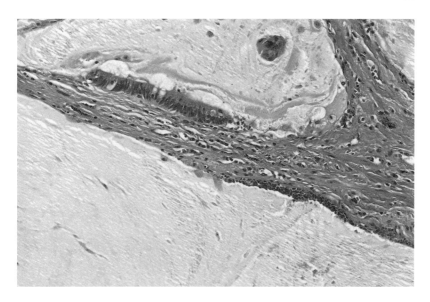

Fig. 45. *Mucinous ("colloid") adenocarcinoma.* There is abundant mucin within alveolar spaces. Scattered clusters of tumour cells are present within the pools of mucin. Columnar mucinous epithelial cells line fibrotically thickened alveolar walls

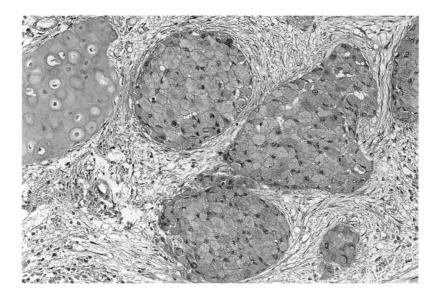

Fig. 46. *Signet-ring adenocarcinoma.* The tumour cells contain abundant mucin within the cytoplasm that pushes the nucleus to the side giving a signet-ring appearance

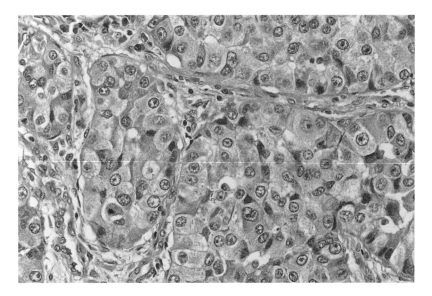

Fig. 47. *Large cell carcinoma.* These large cells have abundant cytoplasm with large nuclei, vesicular nuclear chromatin and prominent nucleoli. No glandular or squamous differentiation is seen

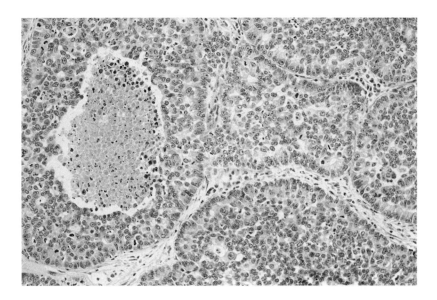

Fig. 48. *Large cell neuroendocrine carcinoma.* Palisading is evident at the periphery of the nests of tumour cells and rosettes can be seen. Necrosis is present and mitoses are numerous

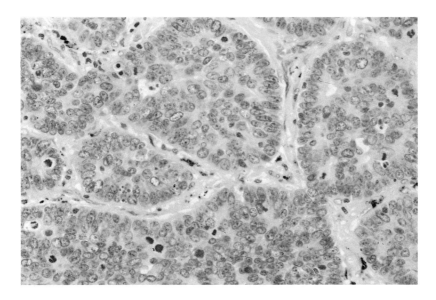

Fig. 49. *Large cell neuroendocrine carcinoma.* Palisading and rosette-like formations are present. Mitoses are numerous. The nuclear chromatin is vesicular and many cells have nucleoli

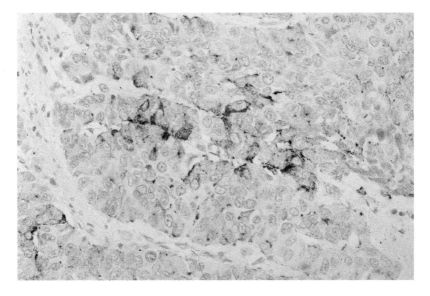

Fig. 50. *Large cell neuroendocrine carcinoma.* Tumour cells stain positively for chromogranin

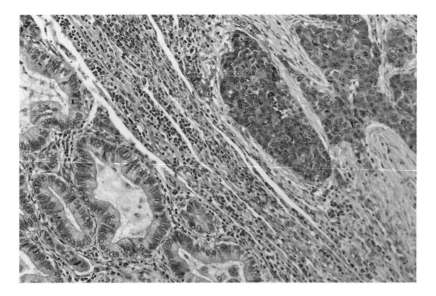

Fig. 51. *Combined large cell neuroendocrine carcinoma.* This large cell neuroendocrine carcinoma is combined with an acinar adenocarcinoma

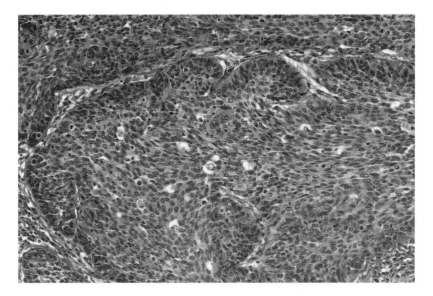

Fig. 52. *Basaloid carcinoma.* Palisading is conspicuous at the periphery of the nests of tumour cells. The cells are hyperchromatic with relatively scant cytoplasm

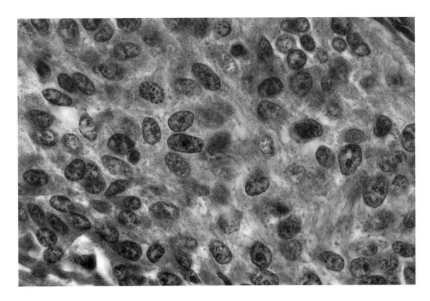

Fig. 53. *Basaloid carcinoma.* The cells have a moderate amount of cytoplasm, dense but coarse or vesicular nuclear chromatin, and frequent nucleoli

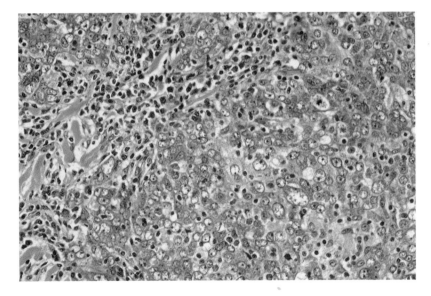

Fig. 54. *Lymphoepithelioma-like carcinoma.* The large tumour cells are intermixed with a lymphoid infiltrate. They have abundant cytoplasm, vesicular chromatin and prominent nucleoli

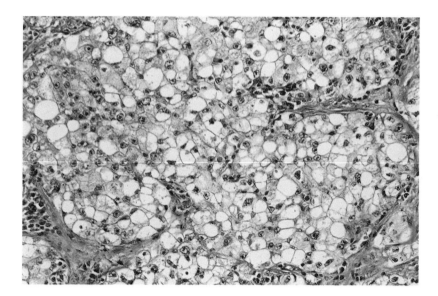

Fig. 55. *Clear cell carcinoma.* These large tumour cells have abundant clear cytoplasm

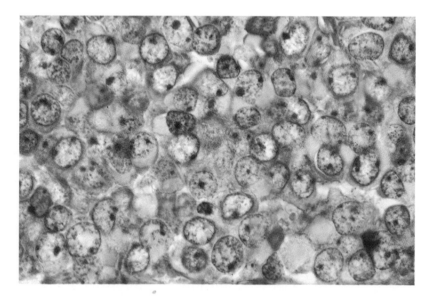

Fig. 56. *Large cell carcinoma with rhabdoid phenotype.* These tumour cells have large globular eosinophilic cytoplasmic inclusions. The nuclear chromatin is vesicular and nucleoli are prominent

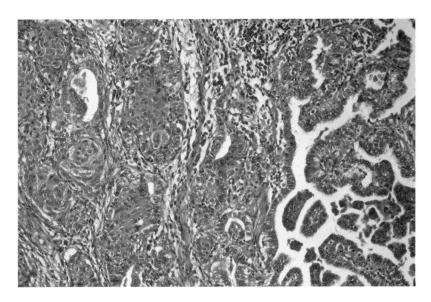

Fig. 57. *Adenosquamous carcinoma.* The tumour consists of squamous cell carcinoma (*left*) and papillary adenocarcinoma (*right*)

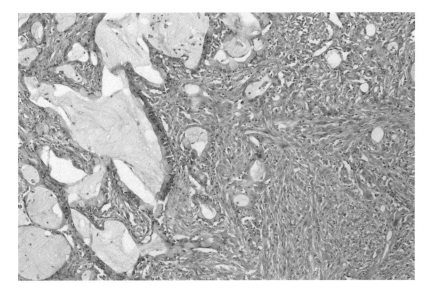

Fig. 58. *Pleomorphic carcinoma.* The tumour consists of a mucinous adenocarcinoma (*left*) and spindle cell carcinoma (*right*)

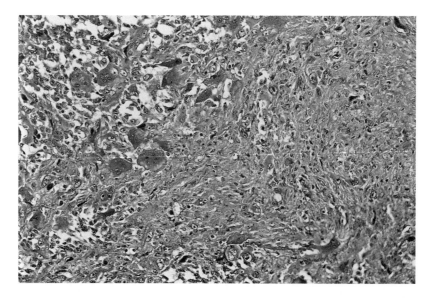

Fig. 59. *Pleomorphic carcinoma.* The tumour has a mixture of giant cell carcinoma (*left*) and spindle cell carcinoma (*right*)

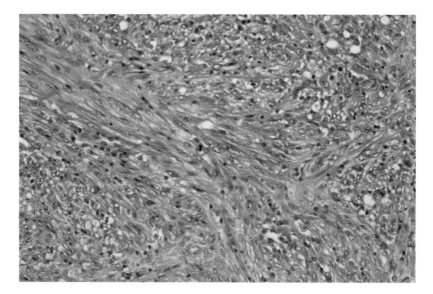

Fig. 60. *Pleomorphic carcinoma.* The spindle cell component shows cytologic atypia but epithelioid morphology

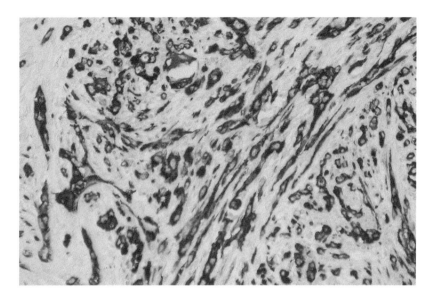

Fig. 61. *Pleomorphic carcinoma.* The spindle cells stain strongly with immunohisto-chemistry for keratin

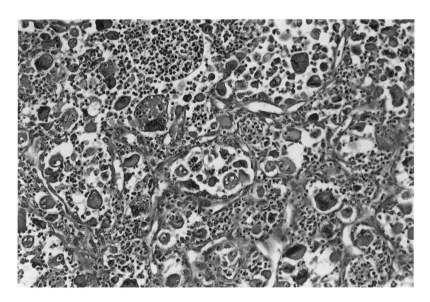

Fig. 62. *Giant cell carcinoma.* The tumour consists of numerous giant cells, some of which are multinucleated

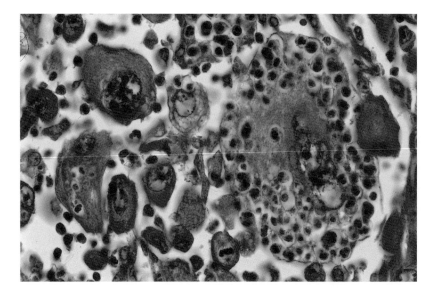

Fig. 63. *Giant cell carcinoma.* The tumour cells are very large with abundant cytoplasm and large, atypical hyperchromatic nuclei. There is a prominent infiltrate of neutrophils, some of which permeate the tumour cell cytoplasm (emperipolesis)

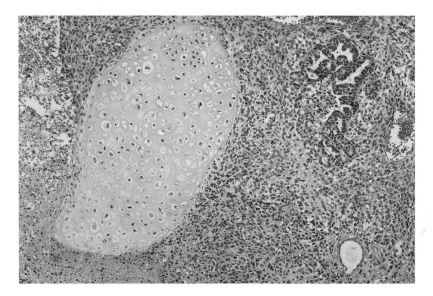

Fig. 64. *Carcinosarcoma.* This tumour consists of malignant cartilage or chondrosarcoma (*left*) and malignant glands or adenocarcinoma (*top right*)

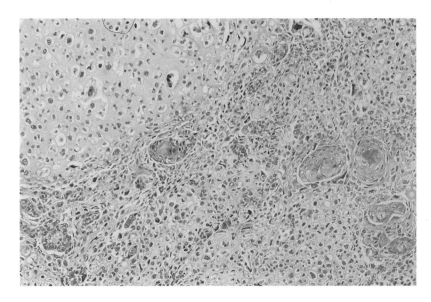

Fig. 65. *Carcinosarcoma.* This tumour consists of malignant cartilage (*top left*) and squamous cell carcinoma (*bottom right*)

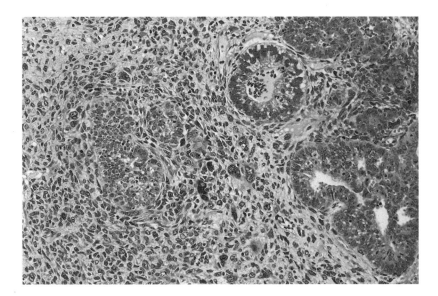

Fig. 66. *Pulmonary blastoma.* The tumour consists of a spindle cell component (*left*) and malignant glandular component (*right*). The glandular component resembles that seen in well-differentiated fetal adenocarcinoma with endometrioid morphology

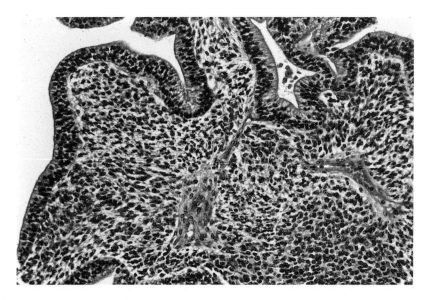

Fig. 67. *Pulmonary blastoma.* The glandular pattern shows the pattern of well-differentiated fetal adenocarcinoma with palisading of nuclei and abundant clear cytoplasm. The spindle cell component has a primitive malignant mesenchymal pattern

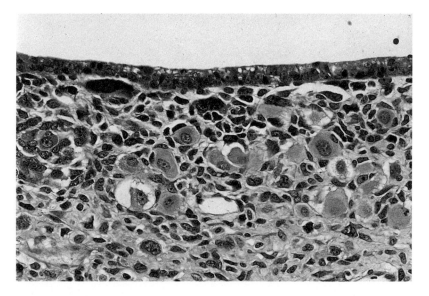

Fig. 68. *Pulmonary blastoma.* The mesenchymal component of this pulmonary blastoma shows rhabdomyosarcomatous differentiation. The cells with abundant eosinophilic cytoplasm indicate skeletal muscle differentiation

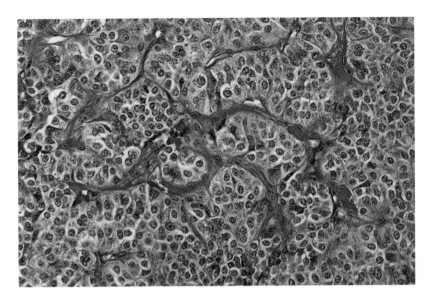

Fig. 69. *Typical carcinoid.* The tumour cells are growing in an organoid nesting arrangement with a fine vascular stroma. The moderate amount of cytoplasm is eosinophilic and the nuclear chromatin is finely granular

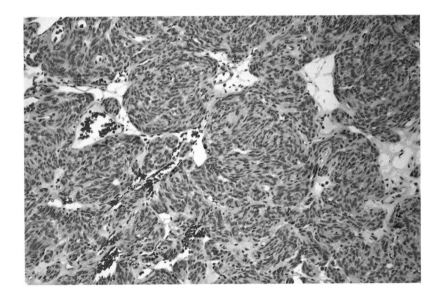

Fig. 70. *Typical carcinoid.* Prominent spindle cell pattern

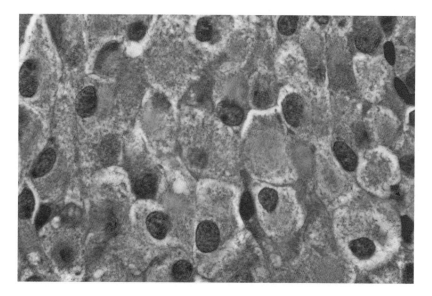

Fig. 71. *Typical carcinoid.* The tumour cells show oncocytic features with abundant eosinophilic cytoplasm

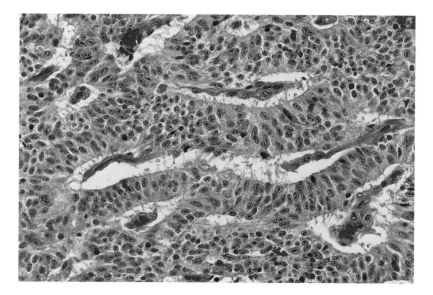

Fig. 72. *Typical carcinoid.* Trabecular pattern

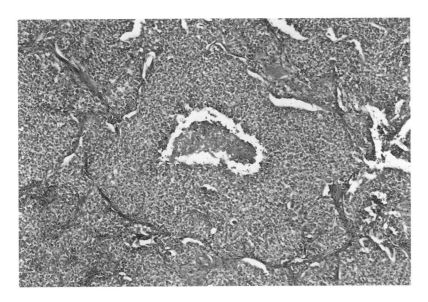

Fig. 73. *Atypical carcinoid.* A punctate focus of necrosis is present within the centre of a nest of tumour cells

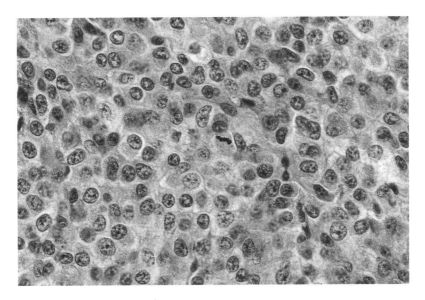

Fig. 74. *Atypical carcinoid.* A single mitosis is present in this high-power field. The tumour cells show carcinoid morphology with moderate eosinophilic cytoplasm and finely granular nuclear chromatin. Nucleoli are present in many cells

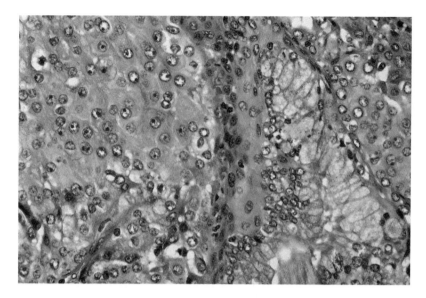

Fig. 75. *Mucoepidermoid carcinoma.* The tumour shows a combination of well-differentiated mucinous glands and squamoid cells

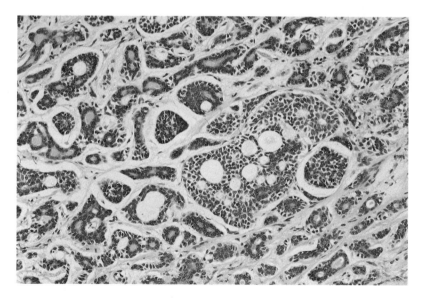

Fig. 76. *Adenoid cystic carcinoma.* This tumour consists of a cylindromatous growth pattern of small basophilic cells with abundant eosinophilic stroma, some of which resembles basal lamina

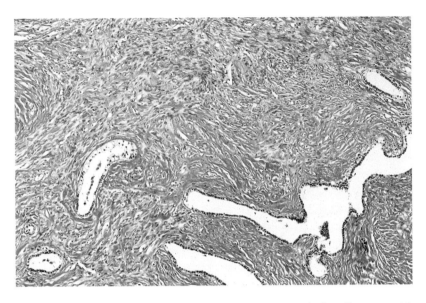

Fig. 77. *Localized fibrous tumour.* The low power shows a spindle cell tumour with slit-like spaces lined by hyperplastic cuboidal-shaped mesothelial cells

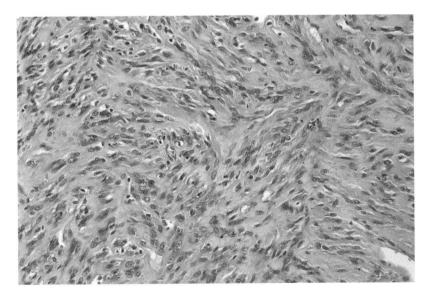

Fig. 78. *Localized fibrous tumour.* The tumour shows round to oval-shaped tumour cells with a ropy collagen stroma

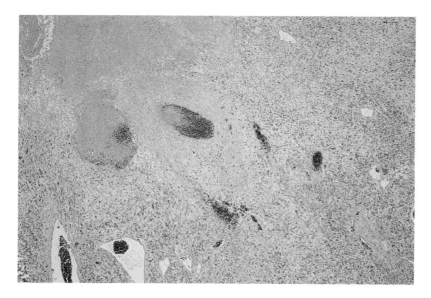

Fig. 79. *Malignant localized fibrous tumour.* Large foci of necrosis are present within this tumour

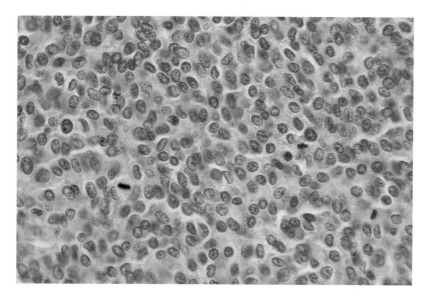

Fig. 80. *Malignant localized fibrous tumour.* Several mitoses are present within this cellular tumour that shows mostly round cells with very little stroma

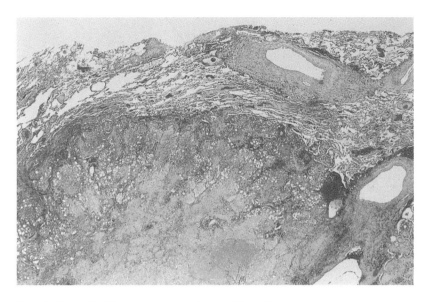

Fig. 81. *Epithelioid hemangioendothelioma.* This nodule of tumour shows increased cellularity at the periphery and abundant eosinophilic stroma in the centre

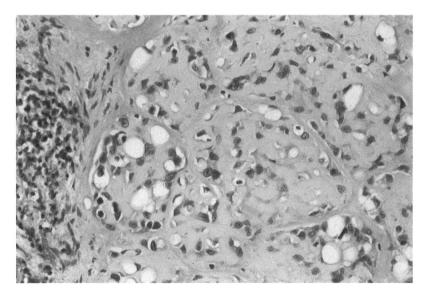

Fig. 82. *Epithelioid hemangioendothelioma.* The tumour shows abundant eosinophilic stroma and the cells have prominent cytoplasmic vacuoles or intracytoplasmic lumina

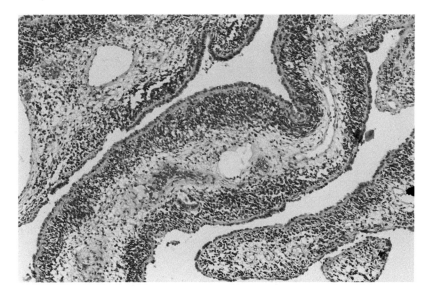

Fig. 83. *Pleuropulmonary blastoma.* A cellular cambium layer is present beneath the hyperplastic mesothelial cells lining the cyst wall

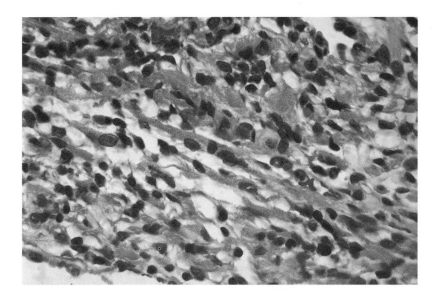

Fig. 84. *Pleuropulmonary blastoma.* The cellular cambium layer consists of malignant cells with abundant eosinophilic cytoplasm, some of which is elongated and shows cross striations

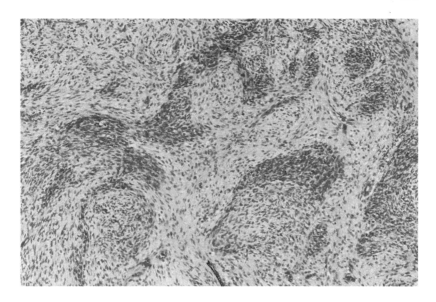

Fig. 85. *Pleuropulmonary blastoma.* The alternating hypercellular and paucicellular pattern is distinctive for this tumour

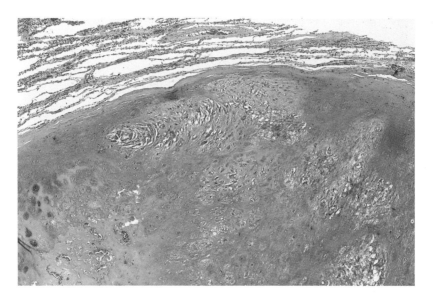

Fig. 86. *Chondroma.* The edge of the chondroma is rounded without the invaginations and epithelial-lined clefts typically seen in chondroid hamartomas. The chondroma shows mature cartilage without atypia

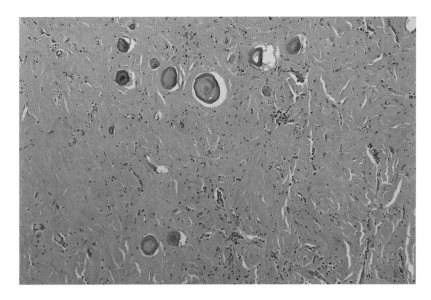

Fig. 87. *Calcifying fibrous pseudotumour of the pleura.* Numerous psammoma-like calcifications are present within the dense fibrous stroma of this tumour

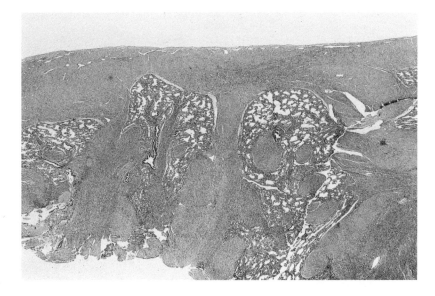

Fig. 88. *Congenital peribronchial myofibroblastic tumour.* There is an extensive infiltrate of spindle cells along lymphatic routes: the pleura, septa and bronchovascular bundles

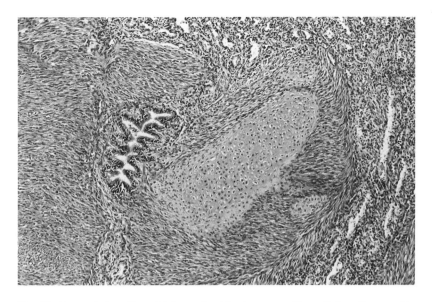

Fig. 89. *Congenital peribronchial myofibroblastic tumour.* The spindle cells resemble smooth muscle cells and infiltrate around bronchial cartilage and epithelium and vessels

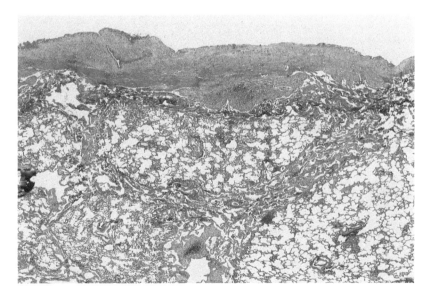

Fig. 90. *Diffuse pulmonary lymphangiomatosis.* The pleura and septa are infiltrated by a proliferation of lymphatics

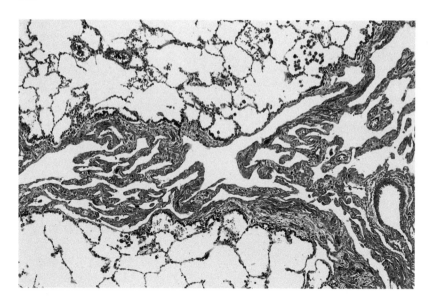

Fig. 91. *Diffuse pulmonary lymphangiomatosis.* The lymphatic proliferation infiltrating along the interlobular septa are highlighted with the trichrome stain

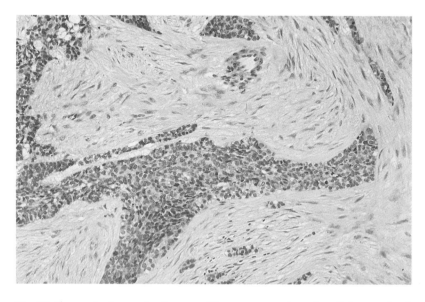

Fig. 92. *Desmoplastic round cell tumour.* The tumour consists of a cellular round cell component within a dense fibrous stroma

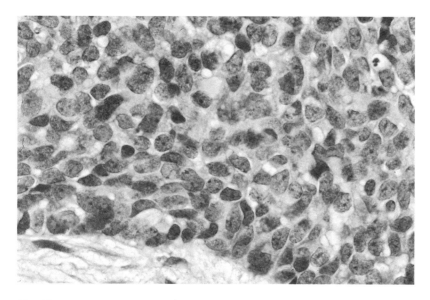

Fig. 93. *Desmoplastic round cell tumour.* The round cell tumour component consists of small cells with scant cytoplasm and hyperchromatic nuclei

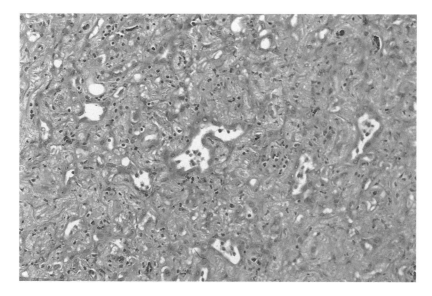

Fig. 94. *Adenomatoid tumour.* Low power shows abundant fibrous stroma with gland-like spaces

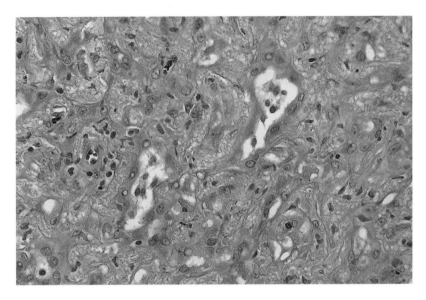

Fig. 95. *Adenomatoid tumour.* Irregularly shaped gland-like spaces are present within a fibrous stroma

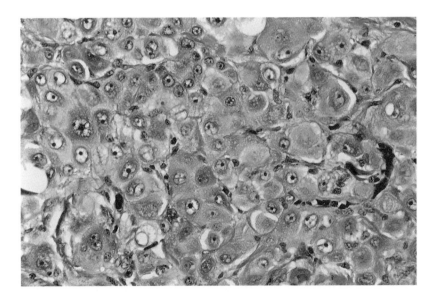

Fig. 96. *Malignant mesothelioma, epithelioid type.* The tumour consists of a sheet of epithelioid cells with abundant eosinophilic cytoplasm and vesicular nuclear chromatin with prominent nucleoli

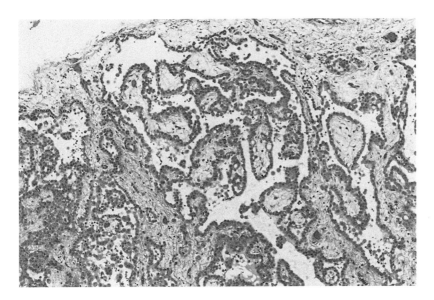

Fig. 97. *Malignant mesothelioma, epithelioid type.* Papillary proliferation of epithelioid cells

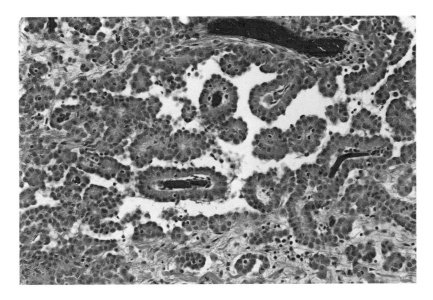

Fig. 98. *Malignant mesothelioma, epithelioid type.* Tubulopapillary pattern

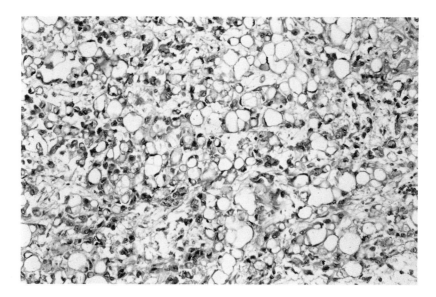

Fig. 99. *Malignant mesothelioma, epithelioid type.* Adenomatoid pattern

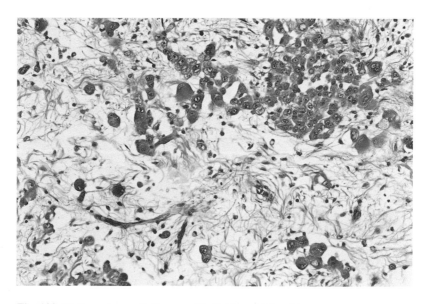

Fig. 100. *Malignant mesothelioma, epithelioid type.* Myxoid stroma

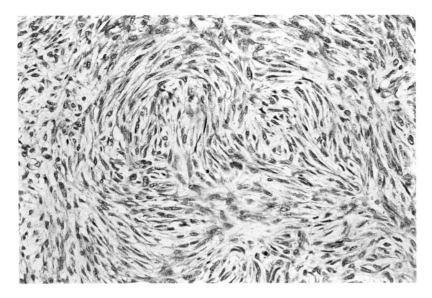

Fig. 101. *Malignant mesothelioma, sarcomatoid type.* Interlacing fascicles of spindle cells

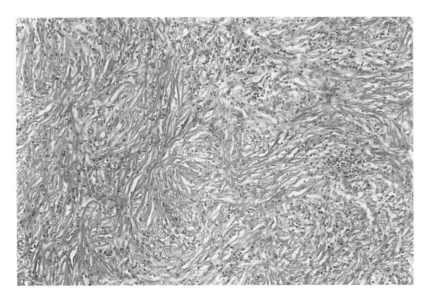

Fig. 102. *Malignant mesothelioma, desmoplastic type.* Storiform pattern of slit-like spaces

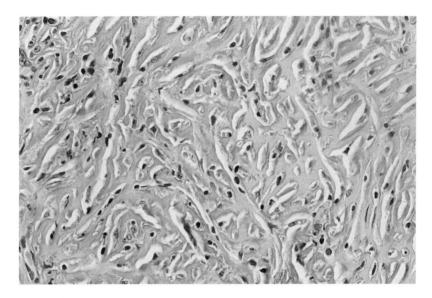

Fig. 103. *Malignant mesothelioma, desmoplastic type.* Haphazard arrangement of slit-like spaces

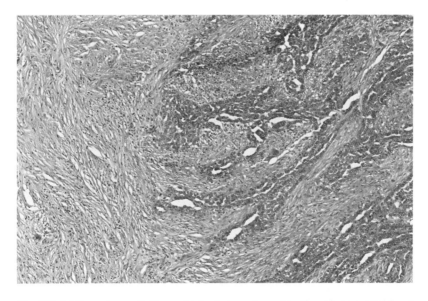

Fig. 104. *Malignant mesothelioma, biphasic type.* A combination of sarcomatoid and epithelioid patterns

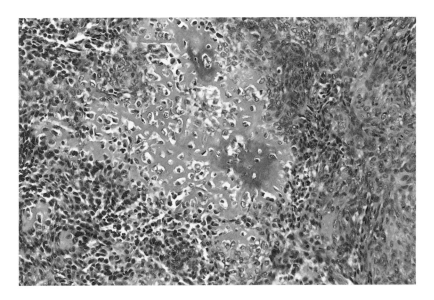

Fig. 105. *Malignant mesothelioma, sarcomatoid type with osteosarcomatous differentiation.* Prominent osteosarcomatous stroma

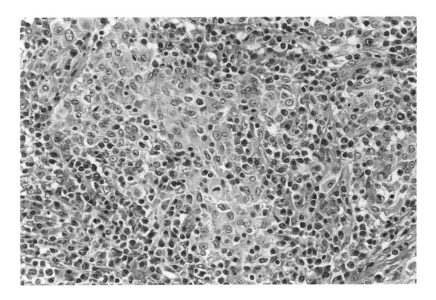

Fig. 106. *Malignant mesothelioma, epithelioid type with lymphohistiocytic features.* A lymphohistiocytic pattern results from the abundant inflammatory cell infiltrate among the epithelioid tumour cells

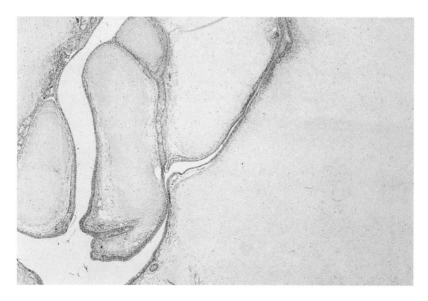

Fig. 107. *Hamartoma.* Lobules of mature cartilage with deep clefts lined by bronchiolar type epithelium

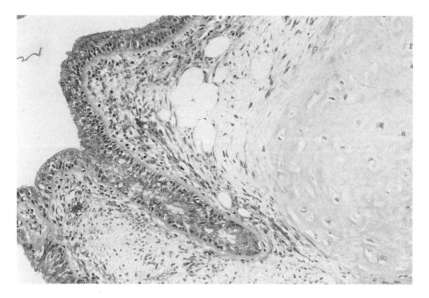

Fig. 108. *Hamartoma.* Adjacent to the cartilage are fat vacuoles and a spindle cell mesenchymal stroma. The cleft-like space is lined by bronchiolar-type epithelium

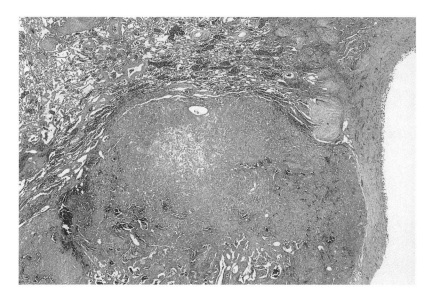

Fig. 109. *Sclerosing hemangioma.* The tumour is circumscribed, but not encapsulated and shows a sclerotic and papillary pattern

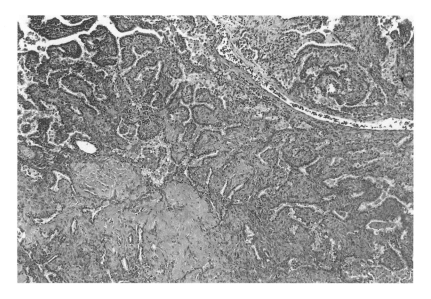

Fig. 110. *Sclerosing hemangioma.* Sclerotic and papillary patterns are present

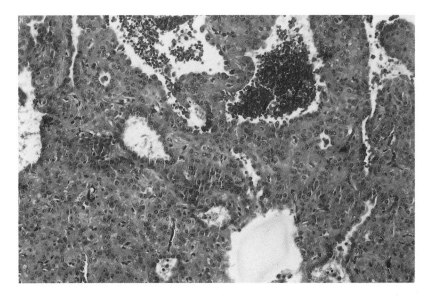

Fig. 111. *Sclerosing hemangioma.* In this haemorrhagic pattern the tumour forms ectatic spaces filled with red blood cells that are surrounded by type II pneumocytes

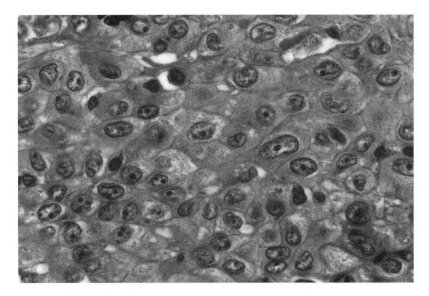

Fig. 112. *Sclerosing hemangioma.* These epithelioid cells are growing in the solid pattern of sclerosing hemangioma

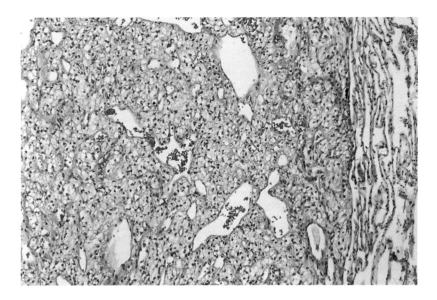

Fig. 113. *Clear cell tumour.* The tumour is circumscribed, but not encapsulated and consists of tumour cells with abundant clear cytoplasm. Sinusoidal, thin-walled vessels are present within the tumour

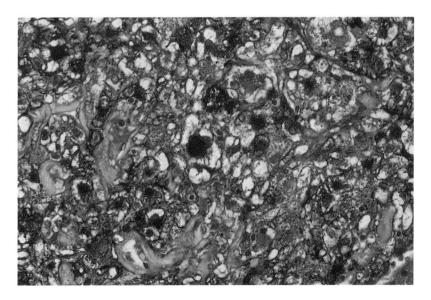

Fig. 114. *Clear cell tumour.* The abundant cytoplasmic glycogen is stained with periodic acid–Schiff

130

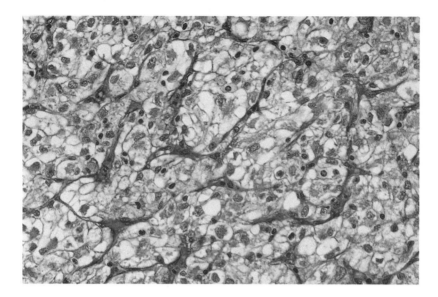

Fig. 115. *Clear cell tumour.* The glycogen is removed in this periodic acid–Schiff stain with diastase digestion

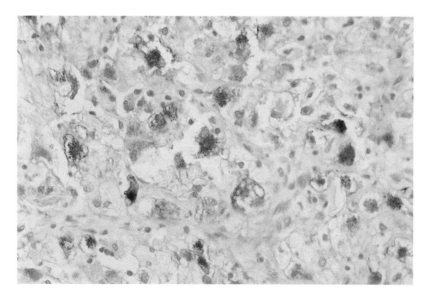

Fig. 116. *Clear cell tumour.* The tumour cells stain positively with immunohisto-chemistry for HMB-45

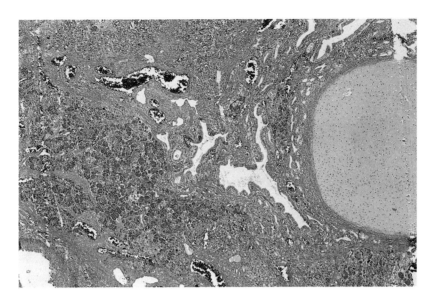

Fig. 117. *Mature teratoma.* Mature cartilage, glands and pancreatic tissue
[From Colby, TV, Koss, MN, Travis, WD (1995) Tumors of the Lower Respiratory
Tract; Atlas of Tumour Pathology, Third Series, Washington, D.C., Armed Forces
Institute of Pathology]

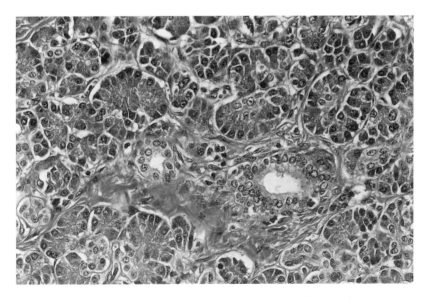

Fig. 118. *Mature teratoma.* Pancreatic tissue with acinar and ductal epithelium
[From Colby, TV, Koss, MN, Travis, WD (1995) Tumors of the Lower Respiratory
Tract; Atlas of Tumour Pathology, Third Series, Washington, D.C., Armed Forces
Institute of Pathology]

132

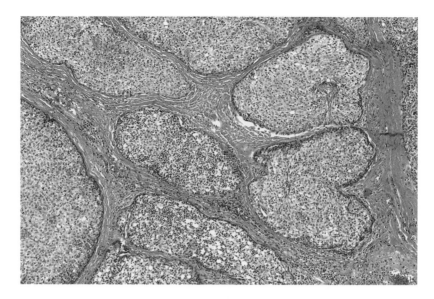

Fig. 119. *Thymoma.* This pleural tumour shows lobules of epithelial cells surrounded by thick bands of fibrous stroma

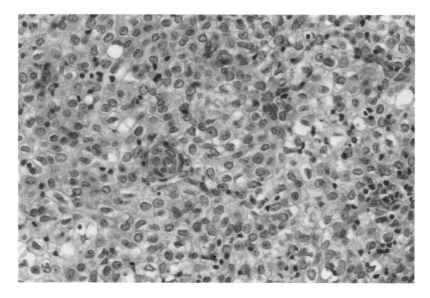

Fig. 120. *Thymoma.* The tumour consists of a mixture of thymic epithelial cells with a few lymphocytes

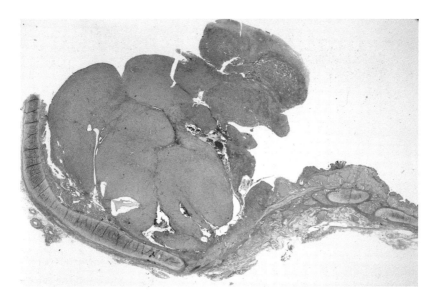

Fig. 121. *Malignant melanoma, primary.* A polypoid endobronchial mass with spread along the adjacent bronchial mucosa
[From Colby, TV, Koss, MN, Travis, WD (1995) Tumors of the Lower Respiratory Tract; Atlas of Tumour Pathology, Third Series, Washington, D.C., Armed Forces Institute of Pathology]

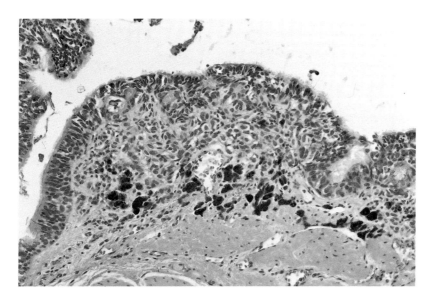

Fig. 122. *Malignant melanoma, primary.* Tumour cells infiltrate the bronchial mucosa and involve the epithelium in a pagetoid fashion
[From Colby, TV, Koss, MN, Travis, WD (1995) Tumors of the Lower Respiratory Tract; Atlas of Tumour Pathology, Third Series, Washington, D.C., Armed Forces Institute of Pathology]

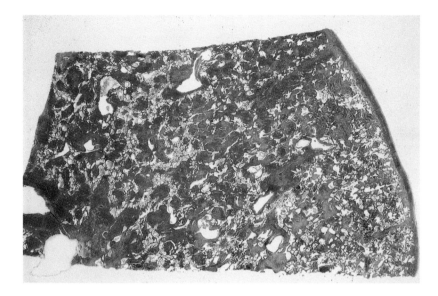

Fig. 123. *Low-grade marginal zone B-cell lymphoma of the mucosa-associated lymphoid tissue.* A monotonous population of small lymphoid cells diffusely infiltrates the lung

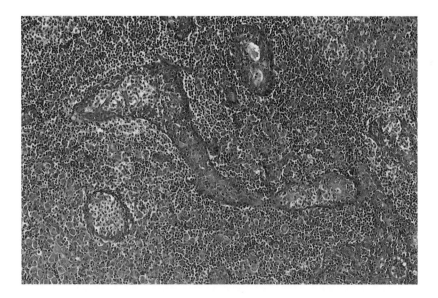

Fig. 124. *Low-grade marginal zone B-cell lymphoma of the mucosa-associated lymphoid tissue.* The lymphoid cells infiltrate the bronchiolar epithelium forming lymphoepithelial lesions

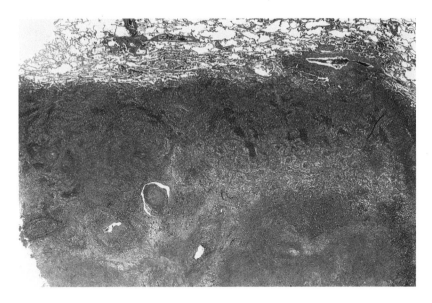

Fig. 125. *Lymphomatoid granulomatosis.* A nodular mass of atypical lymphoid cells shows a large central necrotic zone

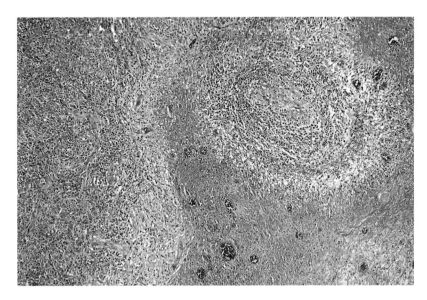

Fig. 126. *Lymphomatoid granulomatosis.* At the edge of the necrosis, the lymphoid infiltrate permeates a blood vessel wall

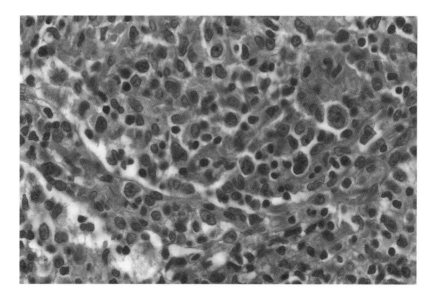

Fig. 127. *Lymphomatoid granulomatosis.* The infiltrate consists of a mixture of large atypical lymphoid cells with medium-sized and smaller lymphoid cells

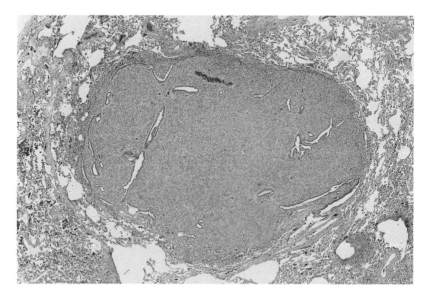

Fig. 128. *Benign metastasizing leiomyoma.* This nodule consists of cytologically benign smooth muscle cells

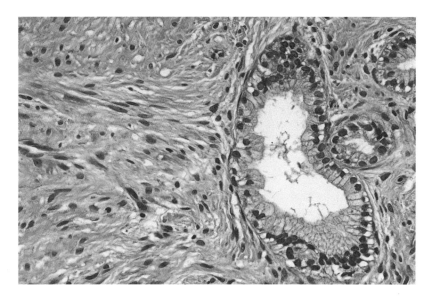

Fig. 129. *Benign metastasizing leiomyoma.* The benign-appearing spindle-shaped smooth muscle cells are associated with hyperplastic glandular epithelium

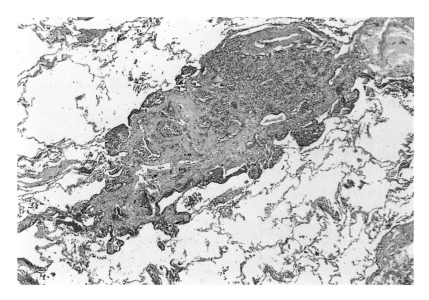

Fig. 130. *Tumourlet.* A small millimeter-sized nodular aggregate of neuroendocrine cells growing in a nested pattern
[From Colby, TV, Koss, MN, Travis, WD (1995) Tumors of the Lower Respiratory Tract; Atlas of Tumour Pathology, Third Series, Washington, D.C., Armed Forces Institute of Pathology]

138

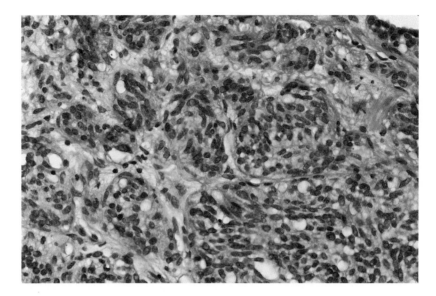

Fig. 131. *Tumourlet.* The neuroendocrine cells have an organoid and nested pattern with a moderate amount of cytoplasm and finely granular nuclear chromatin

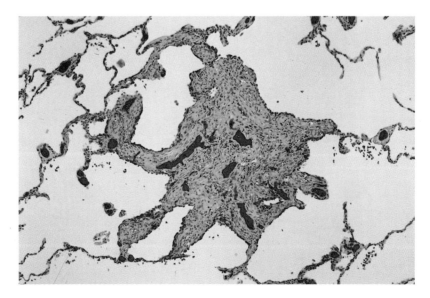

Fig. 132. *Minute meningothelioid nodule.* The lesion consists of a proliferation of uniform cells with moderate eosinophilic cytoplasm in a perivenular location

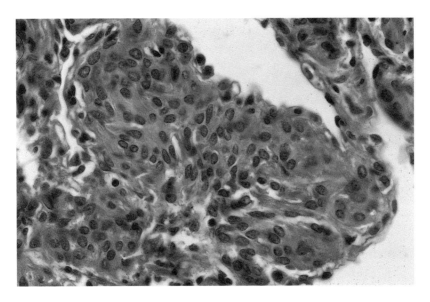

Fig. 133. *Minute meningothelioid nodule.* The tumour cells have an organoid nesting arrangement
[From Colby, TV, Koss, MN, Travis, WD (1995) Tumors of the Lower Respiratory Tract; Atlas of Tumour Pathology, Third Series, Washington, D.C., Armed Forces Institute of Pathology]

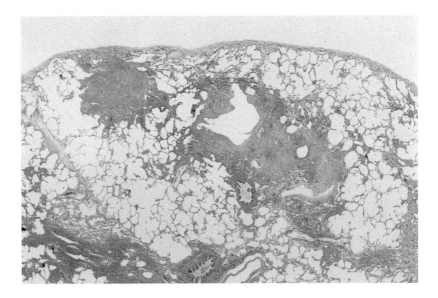

Fig. 134. *Langerhans cell histiocytosis.* Low power shows multiple nodular interstitial infiltrates with focal central cavitation. The edge of the nodular infiltrates shows a stellate-shape

140

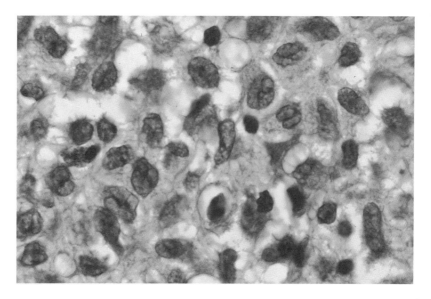

Fig. 135. *Langerhans cell histiocytosis.* The infiltrate consists of Langerhans cells with a moderate amount of eosinophilic cytoplasm and nuclei with prominent grooves

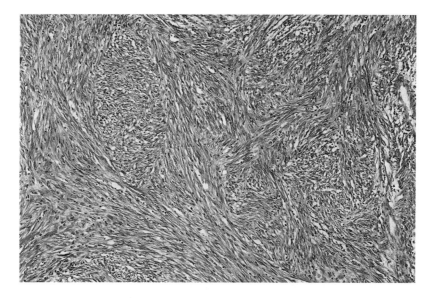

Fig. 136. *Inflammatory pseudotumour.* The spindle cells grow in interlacing fascicles

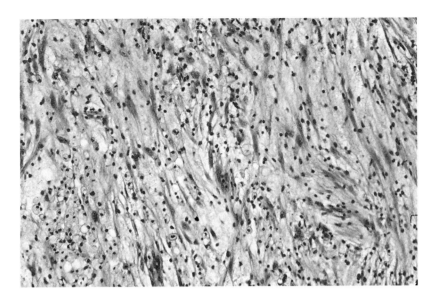

Fig. 137. *Inflammatory pseudotumour.* These spindle cells have a myxoid stroma and mild chronic inflammatory infiltrate

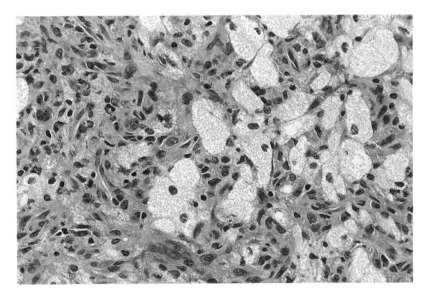

Fig. 138. *Inflammatory pseudotumour.* Numerous foamy histiocytes give this lesion a fibroxanthomatous appearance

142

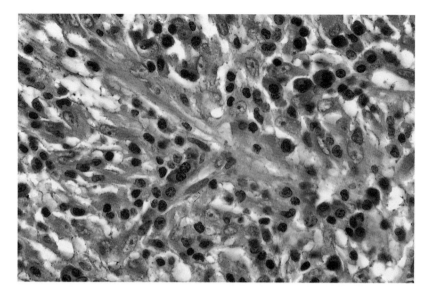

Fig. 139. *Inflammatory pseudotumour.* Prominent lymphocytes and plasma cells infiltrate among the myofibroblastic cells in this lesion

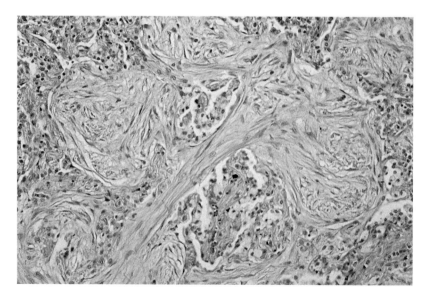

Fig. 140. *Organizing pneumonia.* Within alveolar spaces and alveolar ducts are multiple plugs of organizing connective tissue

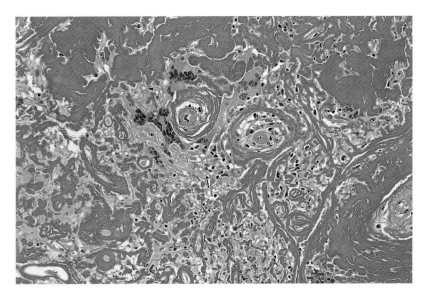

Fig. 141. *Nodular amyloid.* This localized nodule consists of eosinophilic amorphous material with a prominent giant cell reaction

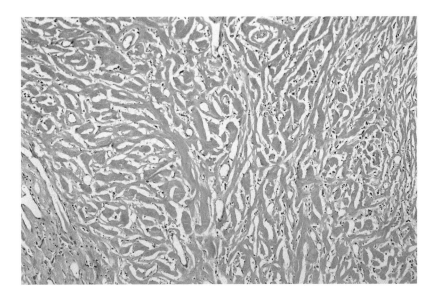

Fig. 142. *Hyalinizing granuloma.* This lesion consists of thick fibrous bands of dense collagen

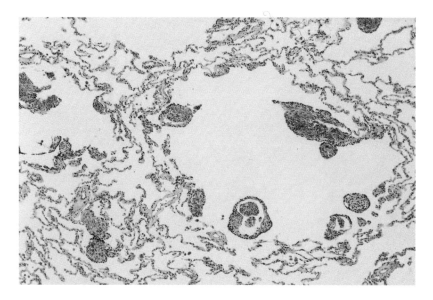

Fig. 143. *Lymphangioleiomyomatosis.* Low power shows cystic spaces lined by nodular smooth muscle bundles

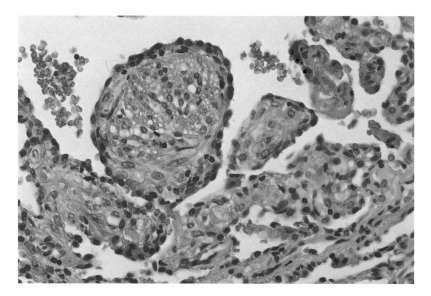

Fig. 144. *Lymphangioleiomyomatosis.* The nodular bundles are composed of round to oval and spindle-shaped cells

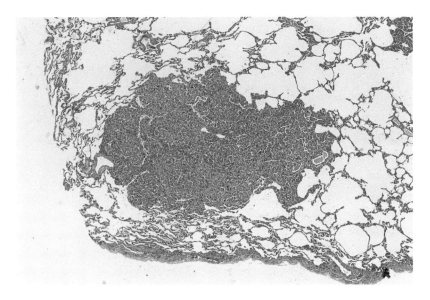

Fig. 145. *Micronodular pneumocyte hyperplasia.* A discrete nodule consists of a proliferation of pneumocytes

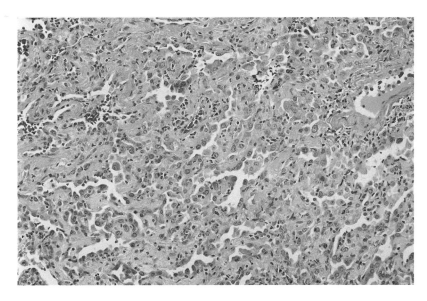

Fig. 146. *Micronodular pneumocyte hyperplasia.* Hyperplastic type II pneumocytes line the alveolar walls that are mildly thickened by fibrous connective tissue

146

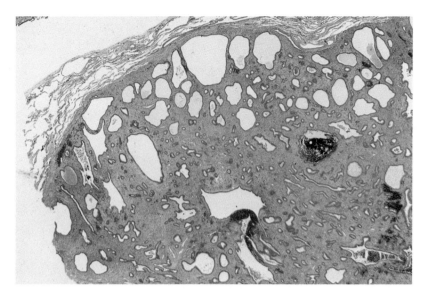

Fig. 147. *Endometriosis.* This case of endometriosis forms a nodular mass or endometrioma with cystic glands

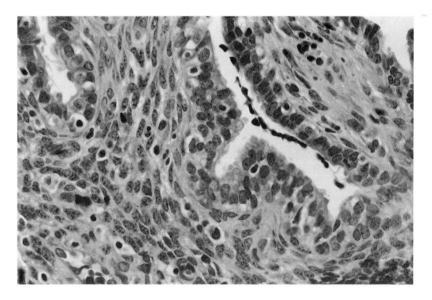

Fig. 148. *Endometriosis.* Characteristic endometrial glands and stroma are present

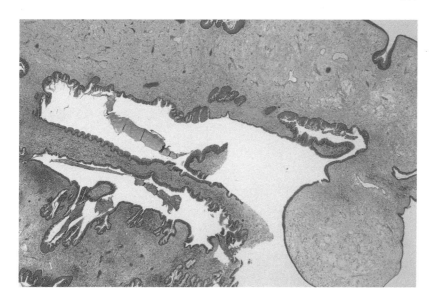

Fig. 149. *Bronchial inflammatory polyp.* This intraluminal polypoid endobronchial lesion is edematous and chronically inflamed

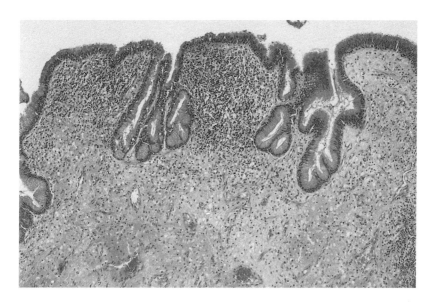

Fig. 150. *Bronchial inflammatory polyp.* The submucosa is edematous and shows chronic inflammation

Subject Index

35 mm Color Transparencies

A set of 200 color slides (35 mm), corresponding to the photomicrographs in this book, is available from the American Registry of Pathology. To order these slides, send the following information to:

American Registry of Pathology
14th Street and Alaska Ave., N.W.
Bldg. 54, Rm 1077
Washington, DC 20306, USA

Or call, fax, or e-mail the American Registry of Pathology Bookstore at:

Phone: 202-782-2666 or 1-888-838-1297 (US only)
Fax: 202-782-0941 or 1-800-278-8513 (US only)
E-mail: bookstore@afip.osd.mil <mailto:bookstore@afip-osd.mil>
Website: www.afip.org <http://www.afip.org> (then go to publications)

Please send me:

_____ set(s) of 35 mm slides of Histological Typing of Lung and Pleural Tumors at $ 150.00 per set.
For Air Mail outside of North America add $ 10.00 per set

Total cost: $ _____.00

Name _____

Address _____

_____

_____

Date: _____ Signature: _____

Telephone: _____ Fax : _____

E-mail: _____

☐ I enclose a check/money order in US $ payable to the ARP.
☐ Please charge my credit card:
    ☐ Visa
    ☐ MasterCard
    ☐ American Express

Card number _____

Expiration date _____

Name as it appears on credit card _____

Prices are subject to change without notice.